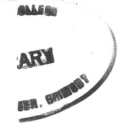

The Handbook of
Ayurveda

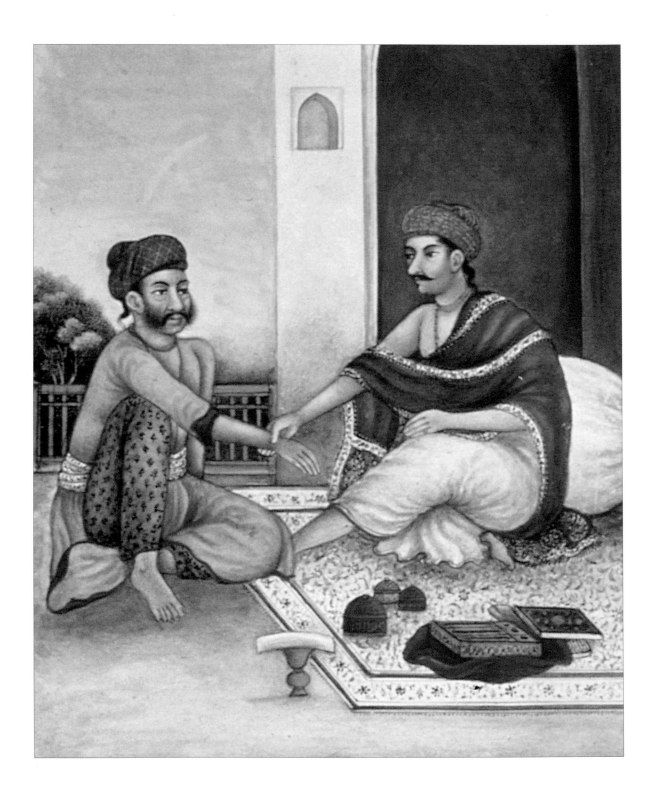

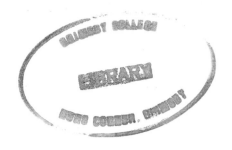

The Handbook of
Ayurveda

India's medical wisdom explained

DR SHANTHA GODAGAMA
WITH LIZ HODGKINSON

"Mind, Spirit and Body hold life in balance with the
three *doshas* like a pot on three supports"
Charaka (1,000BC)

First published in Great Britain in 1997 by
Kyle Cathie Limited
122 Arlington Road
London NW1 7HP
general.enquiries@kyle-cathie.com
www.kylecathie.com

This edition published 2001

Reprinted 2003

ISBN 1 85626 424 6

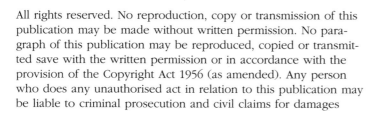

Text © 1997 Shantha Godagama and Liz Hodgkinson
Designed by King & King
Illustration © 1996 Juliet Dallas-Conte
Photography © 1996 Adrian Mott, Katrina Lithgow, Michelle Garrett and Melanie Eclare

Shantha Godagama is hereby identified as the author of this work in accordance with Section 77 of the Copyright, Designs and Patents Act 1988

A CIP catalogue record for this title is available from the British Library

Printed and bound in Singapore by Kyodo Printing Co.

The contents of this book are for information only. It is not intended to be a substitute for taking proper medical advice and should not be relied upon in this way. Always consult a qualified doctor or health practitioner. The author and publisher cannot accept responsibilty for illness arising out of the failure to seek medical advice from a doctor.

Photographic acknowledgements:
Page 64 by permission of the British Library; p.103
    Dinodia Picture Agency, Bombay; p.53 from *Tantra*
    by Philip Rawson, published by Thames and Hudson,
    1973; p.18–19, 84 and 87 by courtesy of the trustees of the
    Victoria & Albert Museum; p.2, 6–7 and 28, Wellcome Institute
    Library, London.

This book is dedicated to the memory of

my mother and my late father and my brother Upali.

To my loving wife, Ranji, for her constant support and

to my children, Suneth, Sumudu and Sujith,

who are studying to be physicians, with the hope that

this book will be of help to them in the future.

To all my lecturers at the

Government Faculty of Ayurvedic Medicine, Colombo

and Professor Anton Jayasuriya,

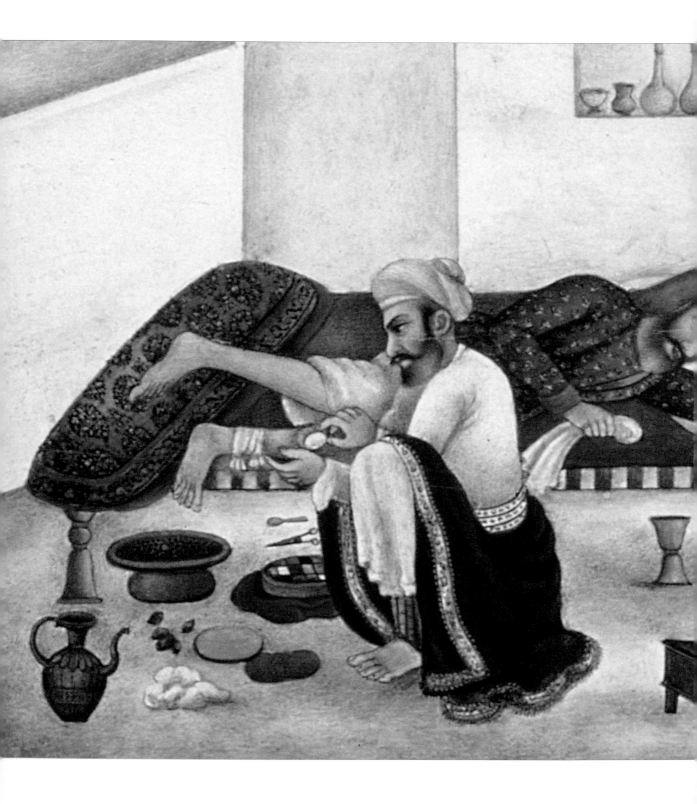

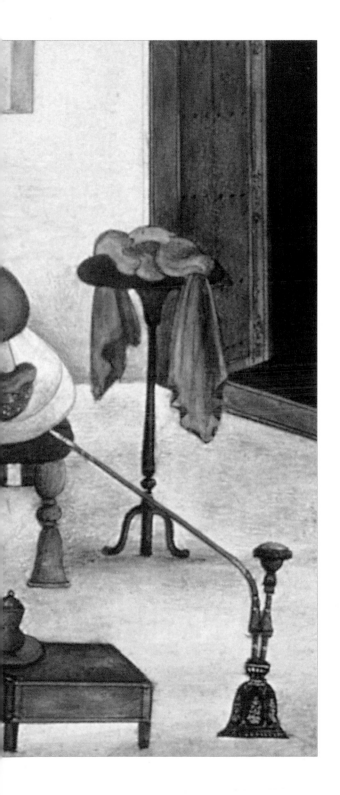

CONTENTS

ACKNOWLEDGMENTS

I am most grateful to Kyle Cathie for commissioning this book. Initially, in the light of my commitments to my practices, at first I believed that the task would be impossible, but Kyle convinced me that a general and, more importantly, accessible book on the laws and practices of Ayurveda needed to be written.

I owe a special debt of gratitude to my teacher, Dr R. B. Dissanayake, former Director of the Ayurvedic Research Institute and the Institute of Ayurveda at the University of Colombo, Sri Lanka and the Commissioner of Ayurveda with the Government Health Department. His help and advice was invaluable. And a special thank you to Sir Maurice Laing and Dr Sidney Rose-Neil. I also wish to show my gratitude to the the late Miss Agnes Hempsell, a yoga teacher and a dear friend who is sadly missed.

Thank you to Annie Allen who spent many hours grappling with my handwriting in order to type up the manuscript. Thanks also to Sue Toff, one of my medical secretaries, who helped me set out some of the more difficult ideas in the book, and to Pamela Anthony who gave up much of her own time to work on the text. I am indebted to my friends Hema Bandara, Irene Nanayakkara, Sreeni de Silva, Shamala Anura Priyanka and Laxman Weerasooriya who have helped me in many ways.

Special thanks must go to Liz Hodgkinson who helped me to rework the structure of the manuscript and present the book in its final form. Her professional manner was much appreciated.

Thanks to Richard Sommerseth for his contributions; to David Grant for the time and effort which he spent editing this unfamiliar subject; and to Kate Oldfield whose excellent, efficient work and good understanding of the subject have helped to bring this book to such a high standard.

Finally, thanks to Teresa Hale, Director of the Hale Clinic, London; Rohit Mehta, Director of the Nutri Centre at the Hale Clinic; Sandeep Garg, Director of the Himalaya Drug Company and Vedic Medical Hall Ltd, London; Gopi Warrior, Director of the Ayurvedic Company and Research Database, London; Dr N. Sathiyamoorthy, Secretary of the Ayurvedic Medical Association UK; Dr Nanda Kumara, Director of the Bharatiya Vidya Bhavan, London; and to Shyla Skears SRN and Mulin Athique SRN, the Hale Clinic *panchakarma* therapists.

AUTHOR'S PREFACE

AFTER PRACTISING AYURVEDA and conventional Western medicine in Sri Lanka, I arrived in the UK in 1979 to be a consultant at the well-known Tyringham Naturopathic Clinic in Buckinghamshire. I trained in Ayurveda for six years at a government faculty, I also studied Western medicine. I spent a post-graduate internship year learning *panchakarma*, Ayurveda's detoxification therapy. Later, I joined a private practice based entirely on conventional Western medicine where I remained for seven years.

Since then, I have witnessed a phenomenal growth of interest in acupuncture. I have also been struck by how popular yoga and meditation, both key aspects of Ayurveda, now are among Westerners. Ayurveda is becoming established in a number of complementary clinics in the UK, and has taken a firm hold in the US, where there are, as I write, already many practitioners and training schools. Increasingly Westerners are becoming interested in Ayurvedic training and before very long, it will become as well-known and well-respected as chiropractic and osteopathy are today.

My aim is to make Ayurveda relevant, understandable and available to Westerners. Most of the material on the subject published in the West has been superficial and offers no more than a partial understanding of this ancient and far-reaching philosophy. It seems to me that, as a growing number of people in the West are becoming disillusioned with orthodox medicine and recognise its limitations, they are ready to embrace the exciting, multi-faceted, holistic approach of Ayurveda.

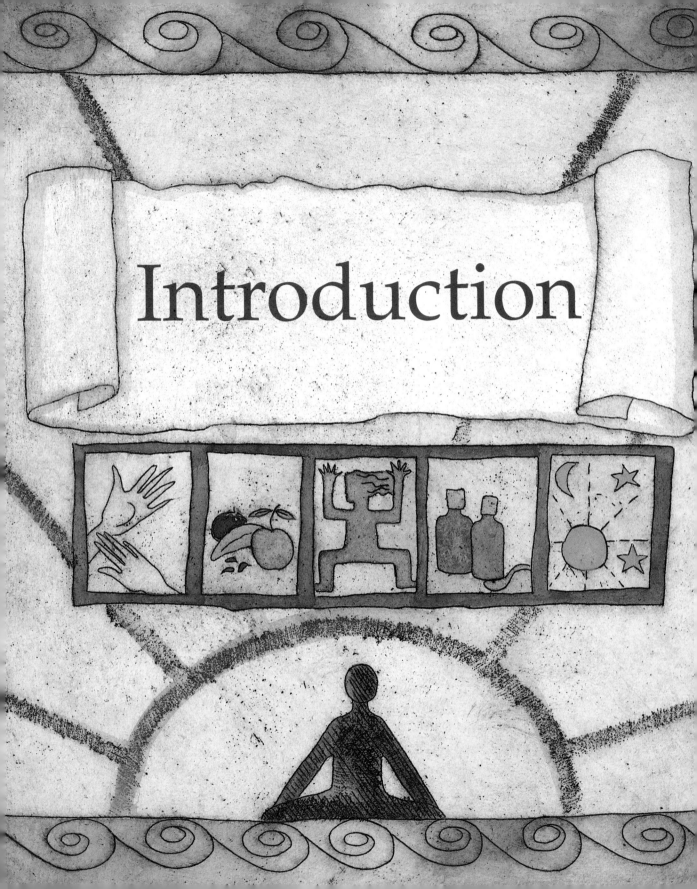

Introduction

The purpose of *The Handbook of Ayurveda* is to explain this ancient, holistic system of medicine in simple terms to those who may have heard of it but know very little about it and would like to learn more. Ayurvedic science, although ancient, could not be more relevant to today's medical challenges and needs. In fact, along with Buddhism, it is the fastest-growing belief system in the West. It is becoming so popular because it complements orthodox Western medicine and, because it understands how and why we become ill, it can offer effective treatment for many conditions for which conventional medicine has not found a cure. The central tenet of Ayurvedic science is that each human being is unique, having a distinct individual constitution, genetic inheritance and predisposition to certain diseases.

TREATING THE INDIVIDUAL

WHEREAS WESTERN MEDICINE has traditionally tended to take the view that all people are more or less the same, and has attempted to treat the condition rather than the patient suffering from it, Ayurveda makes its special contribution by addressing the uniqueness of each patient and by helping the body to protect and heal itself.

Western medicine's view that everybody has the same anatomy, physiology and pathological disease process does not take sufficient account of the differences between people. It also does not usually take the patient's mental attitude into account, nor the state of the patient's mind and spirit. Although the patient has access to psychologists and psychiatrists, they operate separately from the doctors that treat physical conditions and, except for those suffering from what are called psychosomatic illnesses, sick people are considered to require treatment for a physical or mental disorder.

Body and mind

Ayurveda's approach is quite different. It teaches that all illnesses affect the body *and* the mind, and those should never be treated in isolation from one another. Anything which affects the mind affects the body, and vice versa.

Ayurvedic teaching ranges from the relatively simple to the profound, from herbal remedies for such common disorders as coughs, colds and rashes to the belief that, when we are born, we may bring disease processes with us from previous lives. Although founded in a belief in reincarna-

tion, this is perhaps not completely out of harmony with the geneticist's explanation for why every human being is born with particular physical and psychological characteristics, and, more importantly in this context, a predisposition towards certain diseases and disabilities.

A wide-ranging system

Ayurveda embraces medical science, philosophy, psychology, spiritual understanding, as well as astrology and astronomy. It was the first belief system to place deep importance on individual sexuality. (*The Kama Sutra*, an ancient Sanskrit treatise on the art of love and sexual technique, is a Vedic text.) It is based on the accumulated knowledge and understanding of centuries, and recommends yoga and meditation to combat stress-related illnesses.

At the same time, Ayurveda is very up-to-date. It offers practical and effective treatment for many of today's troubling and little-understood disorders, such as ME (myalgic encephalomyelitis, the so-called 'yuppie flu'), IBS (irritable bowel syndrome), depression and hypertension. It is the most ancient codified system of medicine known, yet clinical trials, using present-day scientific methods, are being carried out at major Ayurvedic institutions throughout the world as the search continues for treatments which are effective but do not have harmful or undesirable side-effects. Ancient wisdom has been verified using modern technology. The Ayurvedic Foundation, based in London, holds a database all of the world's most up-to-date research findings (*see* pages 112–13).

Ayurveda is no fossilised, folklore-based

medicine, but a relevant, dynamic, highly sophisticated and advanced system which can meet the needs of demanding Western patients. It advocates herbal remedies but is much more than a simple herbal therapy. It has elements of traditional Chinese medicine, acupuncture and homeopathy, but goes far beyond any one of those therapies alone, encompassing psychology, genetics, sexuality, diet and relationships, and it recommends a personally tailored lifestyle for happy and purposeful living.

No harmful side-effects

Ayurvedic practitioners obey the ancient medical injunction to do no harm. Although the remedies they prescribe are highly effective, none has adverse side-effects and all are made from natural substances and are non-toxic. No artificial materials, or chemicals concocted in a laboratory are used.

In order to benefit from Ayurveda, patients do not have to subscribe to the spiritual beliefs on which it is founded. All they need to do is come with an open mind and a genuine wish to be healed. Although not fully accepted in the West as an authentic branch of medicine, Ayurveda is presently viewed (albeit with a degree of scepticism) by orthodox practitioners as complementary medicine, and clinics are proliferating. It is popular because it works, and it works with, rather than against, Western medicine.

Panchakarma therapy, a unique method of complete detoxification, is, Ayurvedic practitioners believe, the most effective system ever developed for the management and prevention of disease. In the UK, it has been called 'the sleeping giant of complementary medicine'.

In India and Sri Lanka, where Ayurveda is still the principal system of medicine practised, training is now very rigorous. It was not always so, but now Ayurveda advances with Western medical training and the level of entry qualification is constantly rising. And there is progressively more material to study. Six years of study and training at university level are followed by a year's internship in an Ayurvedic hospital. Students have to acquire a substantial knowledge of Sanskrit, the language in which the original Ayurvedic texts were written, just as Western medicine used to be expressed in Latin, and on which all current terminology is based.

Future generations will find it difficult to ignore Ayurvedic medicine and the philosophy underlying it, which will remain unchanged for generations to come. This book is an introduction to and a summary of a system which could fill volumes.

WHAT IS AYURVEDA?

PUT SIMPLY, AYURVEDA (a Sanskrit word meaning the 'science' or 'wisdom of life') is an ancient philosophy based on a deep understanding of eternal truths about the human body, mind and spirit. Unlike orthodox medicine, it is not based on the frequently changing findings of specific research projects, but rather on permanent, wise, eternal principles of living.

Although it originated in the East several thousand years ago, Ayurveda could not be more appropriate for present-day Western society, where so many people suffer from stress-related conditions which conventional medicine has been unable to remedy. It is the oldest healing system known and also the most complete. Its logical, comonsense approach to health and living is combined with philosophy, psychology and spiritual guidance.

Ayurveda has an armoury of physical treatments, from medication to massage, yoga, cleansing and detoxification programmes, and remedies for such disorders as infertility, impotence, arthritis, hypertension, gastro-intestinal problems, chronic illnesses and infectious diseases. It offers natural, herbal remedies which counteract imbalances in the body and can successfully treat most health problems encountered in the West today. Ayurveda does not treat cancer, but it is believed that following the Ayurvedic lifestyle can reduce the risk of contracting the disease. It also offers counselling for a range of conditions, advocates meditation and has recommendations for harmonious living and good relationships.

The eight branches of Ayurveda

There are eight branches, or medical specialities, in Ayurveda (see box opposite).

In modern practice, surgery is better left to orthodox Western medical science. While Ayurvedic doctors used to carry out surgical procedures, it is now conceded that Western techniques are superior.

At the heart of Ayurveda lies the understanding that everything is One, that is everything exists in relation to something else and not in isolation. Western thought has, by contrast, tended to consider subjects of study as distinct and unconnected with other things. When it comes to med-

---

THE EIGHT BRANCHES OF AYURVEDA

- ◆ general medicine
- ◆ toxicology
- ◆ aphrodisiacs
- ◆ ENT
- ◆ paediatrics
- ◆ spirituology
- ◆ geriatrics
- ◆ surgery

---

ical treatment, therefore, the overriding aim is to re-establish harmony between aspects of a person's life which should be, but are not, in a proper balance.

Ayurveda teaches that the body affects the mind and vice versa, that thought processes have physical effects and that disorders of the body cause psychological problems too. There is no such thing, in Ayurvedic practice, as a purely physical or a purely psychological complaint. The two cannot be separated. All matter, organic and inorganic, exists according to a set of pre-determined laws: there is little anarchy in nature. Animals live according to a set of rules which promote their healthy survival and they reproduce in the correct season. The lives of plants follow a pattern that ensures that leaves, flowers and fruits grow in a specific order and no other. Similarly, if humans do not live their lives according to the right principles, and those lives are disordered and chaotic, instead of calm and serene, illness is the result. But, to obey the rules, it is first necessary to know what they are.

Ayurveda lays down a number of principles designed to establish and maintain harmony in body, mind and spirit, and with the world outside the self. If any of these rules is broken, the physical or mental disorder that we call 'illness' results. Just as Judaism and Christianity have the Ten Commandments, Ayurveda, enriched by Buddhist teaching, proposes five principles (see the box below).

Refrain from killing

In the light of the first of these principles, Ayurvedic medical treatments are normally vegetarian. Ayurvedic belief holds that humans are the guardians of all living things therefore killing another living creature is considered wrong. It is believed that the act of killing is a crime which will cause suffering in the killer's *karmic* cycle. In exceptional cases, when a patient suffering from a wasting disease cannot otherwise get the right kind of protein, an Ayurvedic doctor may prescribe meat as part of the recommended diet. Ayurveda is opposed to all blood sports.

Refrain from stealing and lying

Stealing and telling lies both induce fear in the thief and the liar. Not only is it inherently wrong to commit these actions as it will cause others to suffer, but also the fear

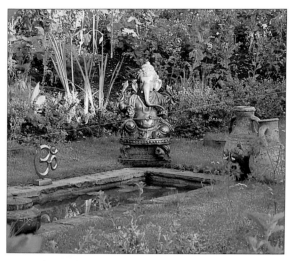

Ganesh symbolises health and protection.

of being found out will upset the constitution of the perpetrator. Ayurveda teaches that it is always wise to consider the happiness of others and act accordingly.

Refrain from sexual misconduct

In its strictest interpretation, the admonition to refrain from sexual misconduct refers to any activity which is not monogamous, faithful and heterosexual and which can cause anxiety, fear and disquiet and can, therefore, result in physical illness.

In most societies, sex was traditionally considered to be a natural biological function for the procreation of the species. Overindulgence and any 'wasteful' activity, such as homosexuality, masturbation, oral or anal sex, cannot produce healthy children and were proscribed in ancient India, where Ayurveda originated, just as much as anywhere else. In today's more liberal atmosphere, when heterosexuality, chastity before marriage and fidelity are less rigidly laid down as rules, a modern Ayurvedic

---

FIVE PRINCIPLES OF CONDUCT

✦ refrain from killing (any form of animal or insect life)
✦ refrain from stealing
✦ refrain from sexual misconduct
✦ refrain from telling lies
✦ refrain from consuming alcohol

---

practitioner would be more likely to advise patients to refrain from any sexual activity which has the potential to harm or exploit another person or even oneself. It is widely accepted that promiscuity may lead to the contracting of sexually transmitted and stress-related diseases. Ayurveda recognises that individuals have different sex drives, and it has to be acknowledged that when Ayurveda was first codified, sexual activity was understood to relate only to men. Women were thought to be passive and not to have their own sex drive.

Refrain from consuming alcohol

Alcohol is regarded as *tamasic* (see page 61) and is not usually recommended as it is harmful to the body and mind. When Ayurvedic texts were being written, alcohol was more or less the only stimulating or intoxicating beverage available. Now there is coffee – the world's most popular drink – along with artificially concocted substances such as lemonade, colas and other soft drinks. To the Ayurvedic practitioner, these are no more desirable than alcohol and, for some people in particular circumstances, alcohol in moderation may be recommended.

Moderation in all things

Ayurveda does not advocate extreme asceticism but rather the Buddhist doctrine of 'the middle road', or moderation in all things. It is worse to suppress emotions and urges than to give expression to them. To maintain good health and a pure spirit we are advised to follow the eight basic tenets of Buddhism, 'the noble eight-fold path' (see the box opposite).

THE EIGHTFOLD PATH OF BUDDHISM

- right understanding
- right concentration
- right livelihood
- right mindfulness
- right action
- right thought
- right effort
- right speaking

We should also adhere to the Ayurvedic rules for healthy living: resist negative thoughts; abstain from verbal abuse; abstain from physical abuse; do not give in to greed; do not give in to sorrow; resist fear; do not let anger persist; shun pride, arrogance and ego.

Causes of the disease process

The disease process may be triggered by a number of causes: evil spirits (this notion has enjoyed a revival with research into 'multiple personality disorder'); poisons and toxins; harmful gases (environmental pollution); fire and accidents; planetary influence (astrology); acts of God (earthquakes, volcanoes, hurricanes, etc.).

In addition to the illnesses and disorders caused by external factors there are two other categories – those caused by an imbalance of the *doshas* (*vata, pitta* and *kapha,* see page 25) and those attributable to mental imbalance.

In classic Ayurvedic teaching, some disorders are seasonal (see pages 75–7) and the appropriate treatment will vary from one part of the year to another.

The concept of *karma*

Ayurveda subscribes to the concept of *karma,* a Sanskrit word meaning 'action' or fate'. In Hinduism and Buddhism it is the doctrine that the sum of a person's actions in previous states of existence controls his or her fate in present and future existences; that human life is one of a chain of successive lives; and that the condition of each life is a direct consequence of actions in previous lives.

There are three kinds of *karma* – good, bad and neutral. As it is believed that *karma* is cumulative, that is that it can be 'added to' or 'taken away from' during a person's continuous existence from life to life, it follows that a good action increases good *karma* or decreases bad *karma*, a bad action does the opposite and some actions do neither ('neutral' *karma*). Many philosophers have acknowledged that we cannot always know the consequences of our actions and have attempted ethical systems to accommodate this fact. The concept of *karma* teaches that we cannot escape the consequences of what we do, and that they may not become apparent in the present life, but in a later life.

Ayurveda acknowledges the possibility of *karmic* diseases and may use the term to describe incurable conditions such as Down's syndrome or spina bifida, suffered from birth and possibly the result of actions in previous lives.

Ayurveda teaches that we all inherit characteristics from our parents and grandparents, indeed all our ancestors. Modern genetic research is demonstrating that this is more wide-ranging than was previously realised. For example, certain types of breast cancer, heart disease and arthritis are now known to be inherited conditions, and there is some evidence to suggest that skin disorders such as psoriasis and eczema have a genetic component.

But Ayurvedic practitioners also believe in reincarnation, that the soul or spirit, at death, continues its existence in another physical form. They believe, therefore, that we bring certain characteristics from our own previous lives – these may be physical or psychological and may include a predisposition to certain diseases – and that the quality of life depends on accumulated *karma*. Every human being is unique, Nobody is exactly like anyone else, and this notion is fundamental to the way Ayurvedic doctors treat their patients.

Longevity

It is assumed that most people want a long, healthy and happy life. There are three conditions required to achieve such a life:

+ a balanced inheritance (in other words, choose your parents with care)
+ a good quality of spirit (one free of envy, anger, resentment and ego)
+ a healthy lifestyle and a good diet

The purpose of Ayurvedic medicine is to enable people to avoid serious illness by having a thorough understanding of how we become ill. It has a strong interest in prevention. But when illness does strike, Ayurveda has a wide range of treatments which help the body to heal itself. All are natural, herb-based remedies. In contrast to Western medicine's drugs (concocted in test tubes and subject to the vagaries of fashion), Ayurveda's treatments are ancient and immutable, have stood the test of time, and have no harmful side-effects.

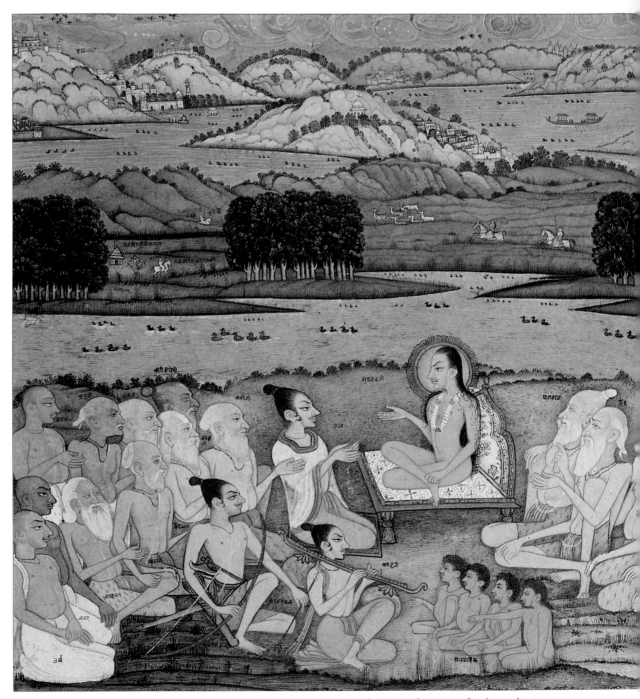

▲ *'Three thousand years ago, humans were affected by diseases. Then some Rishis gathered near the Himalayas to find a solution to conquer disease. They all went into a state of deep*

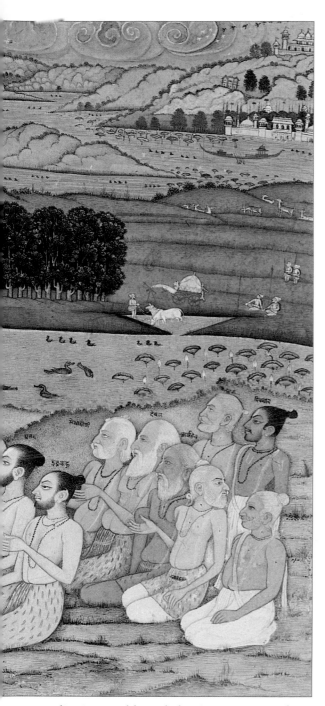

meditation and knowledge was transmitted to them by a supreme god.' (Mahabrama)

A BRIEF HISTORY

TRADITION RELATES THAT in the India of 3,000 years ago, a group of fifty-two wise and holy men left their villages and towns and went to live in the foothills of the Himalayas where they aimed to learn how to eradicate illness and disease from the world. These men, known as the *Rishis*, meditated together and from their meditations they acquired the knowledge which was then codified as Ayurveda.

Subsequently, the Ayurvedic system was written down and was believed to be divinely inspired. The principal text, known as the *Charaka Samhita* and regarded as sacred, opens with a description of the *Rishis'* meditations and forms part of what is the oldest and most complete system of medicine and healing known. When the Ayurvedic texts were being written, disease was regarded as an evil visitation which prevented the individual from attaining self-realisation. To free someone from disease was to enable that person to follow a truly spiritual path, liberated from the constraints of the physical body. A body afflicted by disease resulted in a spirit tied down by worldly concerns and unable to soar. Enlightenment could only be attained by those who enjoyed both good physical and mental health.

According to the *Charaka Samhita*, the *Rishis* elected one of their number, Bhardwaja, to entreat Indra (the Hindu warrior-king of the heavens and a god wise in the treatment of disease) to impart the secrets of health and longevity. Indra was believed to have acquired his knowledge from the heavenly physicians, who in turn had acquired theirs from the supreme god, Brahma. The knowledge acquired by the *Rishis* had three aspects – aetiology (the science of the causes of disease), symptomatology (the study and interpretation of symptoms) and medication. These three components are known as the *Tri-Sootra* Ayurveda.

Hand in hand with Buddhism

Later, the Ayurvedic medical system was augmented by the teachings of the Lord Buddha, who died in about 483BC. Buddhism taught that the mind could be enriched through correct thinking and that following the 'middle path' allowed the mind and the body to survive the long journey of existence, a journey which Buddhist ambition determined should lead ultimately to *nirvana* (a Sanskrit word meaning 'extinction'), a transcendent state in which there is no suffering, desire or sense of self, with release from the effects of *karma.*

Following the teachings of Lord Buddha, more and more Buddhist monks learned and practised Ayurveda in India. There, Asoka, who was emperor of India from about 272 to 231BC, established many Buddhist monasteries and Ayurvedic hospitals, and sent disciples to the Far East and the Middle East (where Ayurvedic practice is known as *Sarak*). So, although Ayurveda has its origins in Hindu belief, it marches hand in hand with Buddhism. And as has been suggested earlier, Buddhism is the fastest-growing belief system in the West.

In Hinduism and Buddhism, existence is believed to be circular (rather than linear), having no beginning and no end. It is, therefore, impossible to pinpoint exactly the origins of Ayurveda as a system, though the written texts can be dated. Ayurveda's followers consider it eternal and permanent. And, though it has its foundation in Hinduism and Buddhism, it is applicable to everyone, everywhere, regardless of their religion and culture.

The arrival of Western medicine

Ayurveda was the principal system of medicine practised in India until the beginning of the 20th century, when it came to be regarded as old-fashioned and 'folksy'. It was gradually replaced by orthodox Western medicine, at least for those who could pay for it. Western surgical techniques, drugs and approach to hygiene swept through India during British rule and more and more Indian students studied and trained in them. Although Ayurveda was never followed by less than seventy-five per cent of the Indian population, sufficient numbers considered it to be out-dated and thus this centuries-old healing tradition was in danger of dying out and it had to fight for its life.

In 1980, the National Congress of India decided that Ayurveda should enjoy equal status with Western medicine and funded many new Ayurvedic institutions. There are now more than one hundred, and their demanding six-year training programme ensures that their Ayurvedic graduates are as rigorously trained as their Western medical counterparts.

Later, the Ministries of Health in India and Sri Lanka set up a Central Council for Ayurvedic Research which would enable proper research work to be carried out using modern scientific methods. These moves have helped to rehabilitate Ayurveda, but it was still virtually unknown in the West until the late1970s and early 1980s. It is now growing rapidly in popularity, partly as a result of the availability of trained practitioners. But there are other, more fundamental reasons for its success.

Since the 1970s, there has been growing interest in the whole range of Eastern therapies. Yoga and meditation are widely taught and practised. More and more people have access to and believe in the beneficial effects of aromatherapy, steam baths, inhalation treatment, massage, herbal therapy, fasting and detoxification – all treatments which have been part of Ayurvedic medical practice for thousands of years.

Limitations of orthodox treatments

Just as significant, people in the West have become increasingly disillusioned with conventional medicine. It may be unbeatable for dealing with acute problems, for putting people back together after accidents and for surgical intervention, but it may perversely be a victim of its own success. Patients' expectations have been raised with every medical advance, rendering all the keener people's awareness of Western medicine's limitations and its lack of success in treating many chronic complaints, a good number of which (most notably stress-related conditions) stem, in part at least, from today's way of life.

We know now, often to our cost, that all long-term medication has adverse side-effects. But this is where the biggest profits lie for the pharmaceutical industry. And modern medicine often fails to address the root causes of many of today's disorders. When infectious diseases were rampant, drugs and vaccination programmes were highly effective and, in some cases, eradicated the disease altogether (in the Western world, at least). Now, Western medicine is relying on the same forms of treatment in its approach to problems which have their origins in mental, emotional or spiritual sickness, and which it simply cannot treat effectively.

A complete system of healing

Because Ayurveda is a complete system of healing, encompassing philosophy, psychology and spirituality as well as a deep understanding of the disease process, it often succeeds where orthodox treatment fails. A unique programme of treatment can be devised for every patient. The approach is never narrowly mechanistic. No two patients, even if they appear to be suffering from the same illness, are the same to an Ayurvedic doctor.

At present, Ayurvedic doctors are not recognised in the West as properly qualified medical practitioners. (Some, including the author of this book, have trained in orthodox Western medicine while training in Ayurveda.) Ayurvedic medicines are officially classified as 'food supplements' and few have a product licence. Yet none has

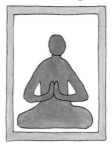

adverse side-effects. The West is now ready for Ayurveda, however. All the elements are there and, unlike any previous or subsequent system of healing, Ayurveda has brought them all together.

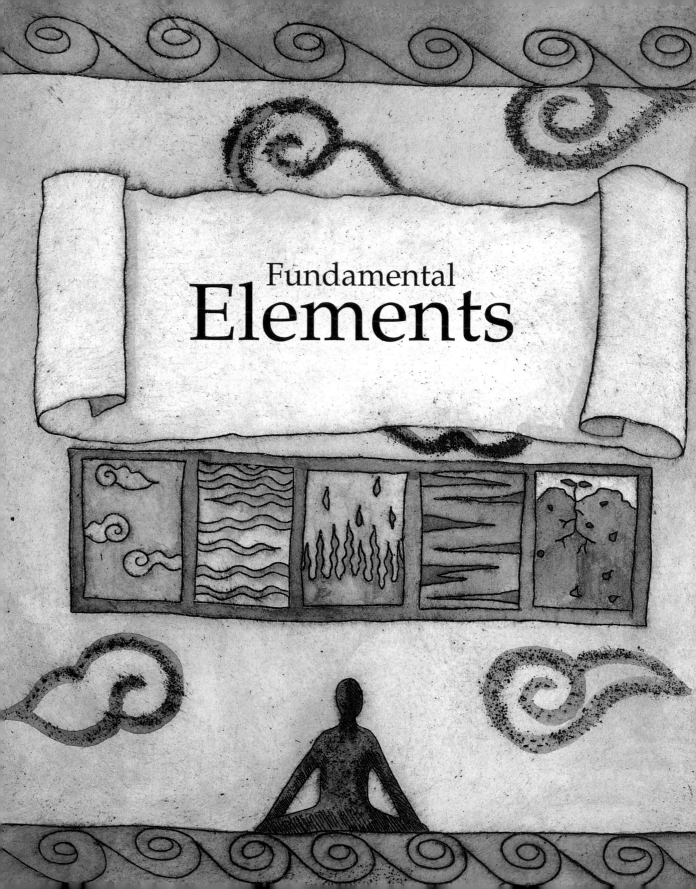

Fundamental
Elements

Ayurveda teaches us that those highly complex organisms we call human beings are made up of a mixture of matter and anti-matter, and that it is the constant interaction between those two which determines the state of our physical and mental health. Ayurveda's most powerful tenet is that nothing function as in isolation and where there is imbalance, the result is illness and disorder. The universe consists of five elements – Ether, Air, Earth, Fire and Water – and the human body is composed of a combination of them. Furthermore, three principal bio-energies – known as the *doshas* – exist in all matter and are composed of different combinations of the five elements. They are called *vata, pitta* and *kapha*. Their influence affects all mechanisms of the body. Most individuals have a predominant *dosha*, which determines body type and temperament.

THE ELEMENTS

IN ANCIENT AND medieval philosophy, and long before the discovery of atoms and molecules, it was held that the world and everything in it was composed of four 'elements' or substances, Air, Earth, Fire and Water. To these, Indian medical teaching added a fifth, Ether. In Sanskrit, the five elements are known as the *mahabbutas*.

Today, in the light of the advance of scientific knowledge, the elements are not interpreted literally but rather as principles informing the nature of existence, metaphors which help us to understand the nature of the universe. Air is movement, setting other aspects of creation into being; Fire is the force which produces heat and light – both essential to life; Water holds everything together; and Earth is matter itself. Ayurveda teaches that the elements pervade every aspect of the human body and that all of the elements can be present in all matter.

Creation from nothing

According to ancient doctrine, the world originally consisted of pure consciousness and was non-material. In time, the lightest element, Ether, was formed from cosmic vibrations. It began to move and its movements created Air. Friction between these moving elements created Fire and the heat of Fire dissolved and liquefied certain elements, thus creating Water, some of which in turn solidified, forming the heaviest element, Earth. This explanation of how the world began may not satisfy Darwinians, Dawkinsites, Hawkingites or other proposers of scientific theories about time,

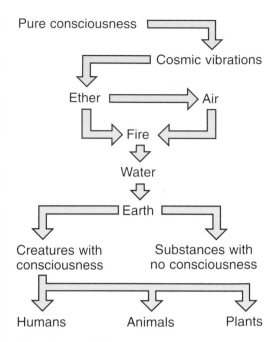

How the world began.

space and the universe. The fact remains that nobody has yet offered conclusive proof of how the world began. The belief underlying Ayurveda is as plausible as any.

Ayurvedic doctrine holds that all organic matter – plants, grains, animals – are formed from the Earth element, which also contains the inorganic substances of the mineral world. Earth gave birth, as it were, to all other matter. It also proposes that all five elements may be present in all matter – Water, when it is frozen, becomes solid like Earth; Fire melts it back to Water; more Fire turns the Water to steam, which disappears into Air and the Ether.

Humans have five senses, which correspond to the five elements. Sound is transmitted through Ether; Air, which Ayurveda teaches is related to nervous system, is believed to correspond to touch; Fire, which we see as light and colour, relates to sight; Water is necessary to taste (a dry tongue cannot distinguish flavours), and Earth is connected with the sense of smell – the nose relates to the excretory organs, (people with constipation often have bad breath and a diminished sense of smell).

As always with Ayurveda, everything ties up with everything else. There is harmony and synchronicity, and it is disharmony. which creates illness. Ayurvedic treatment aims to recreate harmony as far as possible.

THE DOSHAS

AYURVEDIC MEDICINE IS based on the concept of the three *doshas*, or *tridosha*. There is no exact English equivalent of these Sanskrit words, but *dosha* is commonly taken to mean roughly 'force' or 'fault'. So, the *doshas* are bodily energies (sometimes called bio-energies) which influence all living matter and mental energies too. And, because the term also means 'fault', it is understood that any imbalance will lead to a disorder in the body or the mind.

Although the concept of the *doshas* is unique to Ayurveda, it is not unlike the traditional Western idea of three basic body types – ectomorph (lean and delicate), mesomorph (compact and muscular) and endomorph (stocky). Most of us are a combination of two (or all three) types, with one predominant. The three *dosha* types are known as *vata* (the lightest, portrayed by the colour blue), *pitta* (the medium, portrayed by red) and *kapha* (the heaviest, portrayed by yellow). Somebody with dominant *vata* energy tends to be thin, restless

and creative; the *pitta* type mostly conforms to a happy medium; *kapha* people tend to be heavy, slow and lethargic.

Ayurveda teaches that everything in the world is made up of a combination of the three *doshas*, and that the *doshas* themselves combine two of the five elements: *vata* is Ether and Air; *pitta* is Fire and Water; *kapha* is Water and Earth.

Systems of categorisation

Most systems of medicine, ancient and modern, have attempted to divide the human race into types. The older the system, the more likely it is that the categories correspond to forces which are perceived to prevail in nature. In ancient China, *yin* and *yang* corresponded to the passive, female principle, characterised by earth, dark and cold, and the active, creative, male principle, associated with heaven, heat and light. These counterbalanced energies were believed to dominate everything, from the food we eat to a predisposition to certain types of illness. In Europe in the Middle Ages, the humours were believed to be fluids secreted by the body and which profoundly influenced physical type, mental state and behaviour. The predominance of a humour determined a person's nature – if it was blood, the person was deemed sanguine (happy and positive), if choler, choleric (hot-tempered and angry), if phlegm, phlegmatic (slow and calm), if melancholy, melancholic (tending to sadness).

In more recent times, people have been characterised as extrovert (cheerful, positive and outgoing) or introvert (shy and reflective), passive or agressive. The idea

25

that our thought processes are influenced by bodily 'humours' or 'forces' is considered by many to be outdated, but psychologists have not yet conclusively shown what factors determine what type of person we are. As we shall see, Ayurveda offers useful and interesting insights into psychological and behavioural characteristics.

Nature or nurture?

Genetic research has provided insights, but has also fuelled controversy. It is not difficult to accept that we 'inherit' certain characteristics – hair colour, height, the shape of our nose, even a predisposition to certain diseases. But modern psychological theory has tended to the view that our personalities and behavioural characteristics are formed after we are born and cites 'conditioning' and 'environmental factors'. There are, however, those theorists who suggest that it is not only physical characteristics which are genetically determined – 'Is there a homosexual gene?' and 'Are some people born destined to a life of violence and crime?' are questions which stir up furious debate.

Ayurveda has never made this distinction between the physical and the psychological. It believes in both visible and invisible forces and embraces science, medicine, psychology and the spiritual. We are all part of the One, of a whole, and, if we learn to live in harmony with nature (both internal and external), we will enjoy long life and good health.

Ayurveda teaches that each person's dominant *dosha* is determined at conception, when the sperm fertilises the egg. It is determined by a combination of parental inheritance, mental and physical constitution, astrological influence and *karma*. A very small number of people are 'balanced', that is their *doshas* are in perfect equilibrium. Most conform to a 'type', a mixture of two *doshas*, with one slightly more dominant than the other. The prevailing *dosha* determines not only our physical appearance, but also any predisposition to particular conditions or disorders, and how we think and feel. It influences not only our body shape but how high or low our sex drive is, whether we feel happy or depressed, whether we take a relaxed view of the world or worry, and so on. For example, *vata* types are likely to have a high sex drive, whereas *kapha* types may be less ardent but are more romantic. *Vata* people are prone to depression and are worriers; *kapha* people to inactivity and are rarely troubled by anxiety. *Pitta* types manage to steer clear of extremes and are often described as 'the happy medium'. It is important to remember that no individual will display the characteristics of their dominant *dosha* in 'undiluted' form.

The importance of balance

The concept of a predominant dosha is more comprehensive than other systems for categorising people. It affords the most complete and holistic understanding of well-being and illness in all its forms. The *doshas* govern all of the physiological and chemical activities in the body and the aim of Ayurveda is to bring them as nearly as possible into balance – the more balanced they are, the more healthy a person is. *Vata*, *pitta* and *kapha* energies move throughout the body and produce both the

THE DOSHAS AND RELATED PARTS OF THE BODY

Each part of our body comes under the influence of one of the three doshas.

KAPHA
- Sinuses
- Nostrils
- Throat
- Bronchi
- Lungs

PITTA
- Liver
- Spleen
- Gall bladder
- Stomach
- Duodenum
- Pancreas

VATA
- Small intestines
- Large intestines

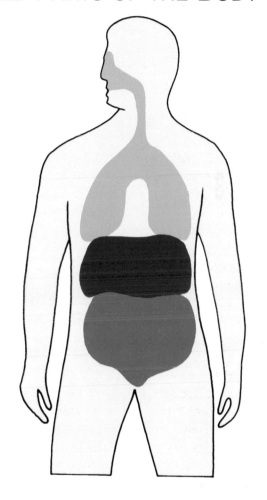

good and bad effects. The role of the Ayurvedic doctor is to assess the effects of the *doshas* and to counter the influence of those which are harmful.

Although the *doshas* cannot be seen, their influence can be monitored. Cells appear different according to which *dosha* dominates (*vata*-dominant cells are very active; *pitta*-dominant cells are fierily active and *kapha*-dominant cells have a high fat and water content). The *doshas* do not lend themselves to scientific proof; but their role and importance has been recognised for thousands of years, they apply equally to men and women, and treatment based on an understanding of them works.

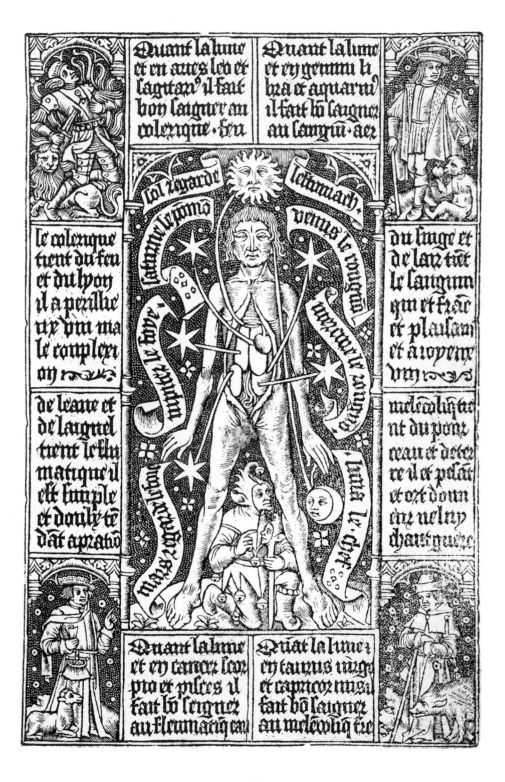

SYSTEMS OF CHARACTERISATION

Ayurvedic bio-energies

+ *vata* – air
+ *kapha* – phlegm
+ *pitta* – bile

Chinese bio-energies

+ *yin* – negative
+ *yang* – positive

The European humours

+ blood
+ choler
+ phlegm
+ melancholy

◄ *The concept of the* doshas *responds to the idea of the four 'humours' (portrayed here with their related organs), prevalent in Europe in the Middle Ages. The humours were believed to be fluids secreted by the body and which profoundly influenced physical type, mental state and behaviour. The predominance of a humour determined a person's nature – if it was blood, the person was deemed sanguine (happy and positive); if choler, choleric (hot-tempered and angry); if phlegm, phlegmatic (slow and calm); if melancholy, melancholic (tending to sadness). Ayurveda believes that everyone's physical and mental characteristics are controlled by three bio-energies, or* tridosha, *known as* vata, pitta *and* kapha.

VATA (see pages 40-1)

THE *VATA* ENERGY is composed of Air and space. It corresponds approximately to the body's nervous system and, in modern terms, *vata*'s functions could be said to be equivalent to the actions of neurotransmitters in the brain. *Vata* controls respiration and elimination, and is characterised as dry, light, rough and quick.

Vata is considered to be the most influential of the *doshas* as it guides all bodily functions and is the main principle of movement in the body. It is connected with activity and vitality, controls the 'empty' spaces within the body (the sinuses, the abdominal cavity, the tracts of the lungs and the inner ear) and the nervous system. *Vata* also controls cell division, the formation of cell layers, and the actions of the heart, lungs, stomach and intestines. It guides the activities of the brain and the motor organs, and is responsible for the elimination of waste matter. An excess of *vata* energy may result in dehydration and associated problems, premature ageing, dry skin and other skin complaints and the slow healing of wounds. An insufficiency of *vata* can result in a feeling of heaviness and sluggishness, and poor circulation.

Vata-dominant types tend to be light in weight, insubstantial, ethereal and creative; they can also be unreliable and changeable. When young, they are usually very thin and athletic, and often display originality of thought. The pure *vata* type is either very tall or very short – tending to one extreme or the other – bony and energetic.

Other features of *vata* types include thin hair and eyelashes, and small eyes. They are

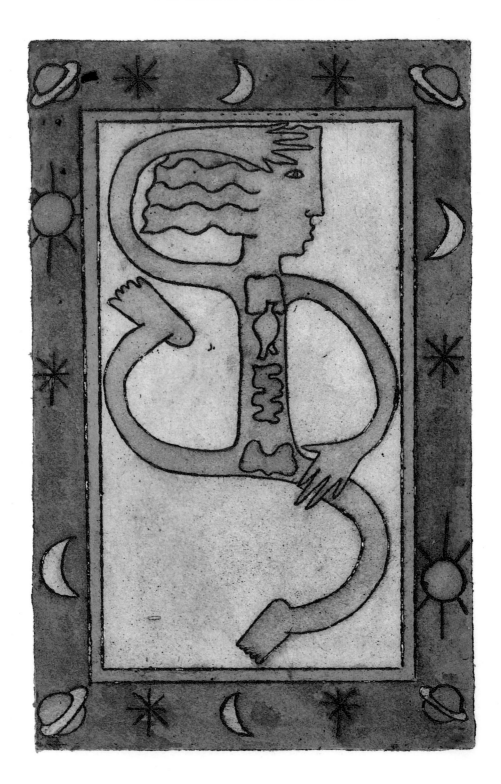

not very muscly and the voice may have a high, thin, cracked tone. Skin tends to be dry. They do not eliminate copiously, have rapid metabolism, enjoy their food (though do not favour rich or luxury foods) and do not gain weight readily. These are quick, active people, always on the go.

Vata people are quick to learn, but often do not retain their recently acquired knowledge. They may be found working in the media where there is a rapid turnover of information. They are prone to anxiety, tension, fear and depression – nature's worriers. They tend towards asceticism and often have a well-developed spiritual side which leads them to study and an interest in esoteric subjects. Some may even have clairvoyant or psychic abilities.

The *vata* pulse is known as 'the snake'. Its rate is 80–100 per minute. It is fast, narrow, feeble, cool and irregular.

The five types of *vata*

There are five types of *vata*, seated (in a loose rather than literal sense) in the body:

praana (the head), *udana* (the chest), *samaana* (the stomach), *vyaana* (the heart) and *apaana* (the pelvis).

✦ *Praana vata* resides in the mouth, head, ear, tongue, nose and chest. Its purpose is to regulate functions such as breathing, sneezing and spitting. An imbalance causes hiccups, hoarseness, coughing and breathing difficulties.

✦ *Udana vata* resides in the chest, larynx and throat. It governs speech, mental attitudes such as enthusiasm and positiveness, physical and mental strength, and the body's colouring. Imbalance causes ear, nose and throat complaints, speech difficulties, and heart problems.

✦ *Samaana vata* resides in the stomach and duodenum. It controls digestion and the conversion of food into waste products, and carries away sweat and water. An imbalance causes indigestion, diarrhoea, gastric ulcers and inflammations.

CHARACTERISTICS OF THE PREDOMINANTLY *VATA* INDIVIDUAL:

- ✦ a thin body and little weight gain
- ✦ rough, dry skin which can crack easily
- ✦ teeth prone to decay
- ✦ small, dull-looking eyes (not always)
- ✦ eating quickly and irregularly
- ✦ erratic memory
- ✦ insomnia
- ✦ restlessness

- ✦ nail biting
- ✦ decisiveness
- ✦ ability to earn money quickly (and spend it just as quickly)
- ✦ difficulty in sustaining relationships
- ✦ high sex drive
- ✦ dreams about flying, jumping climbing, running and tall trees

✦ *Vyaana* vata is present everywhere, but its main seat is in the area of the heart. It is the most powerful *vata* in the body and controls the circulation of the blood. It also governs the formation of sweat and lymph (a colourless fluid), and motor functions. An imbalance causes fever, spasms, high blood pressure, blood disease, and circulatory problems.

✦ *Apaana* vata resides in the colon, rectum, bladder and genitals. It governs urination, defecation, menstruation and the delivery of a foetus from the uterus. An imbalance causes colorectal, urinogenital and intestinal disorders.

Some symptoms of a *vata* imbalance

An excess of *vata* influence may also cause the following symptoms: a darker than usual complexion, furrowed tongue and dry lips, dry eyes, a hacking cough, dark yellow urine and hard, dry, dark faeces. In short, *vata* excess leads to the whole body being dehydrated. There is too much Air and not enough Water.

PITTA (see pages 40–1)

THE *PITTA* ENERGY is composed of Fire and Water. It governs the generation and conservation of body heat, digestion and metabolism, and intelligence. The main seat of *pitta* energy is the stomach.

Pitta-dominant people tend to the medium both physically and psychologically. They have a generally smooth skin and they tend to go grey early, and men go bald prematurely. Pitta types have a strong metabolism and good appetite, favouring bitter, astringent, sweet flavours and cold drinks. They perspire freely and tend to a warm body temperature. They are fairly active, but baulk at hard work. They are sharp, ambitious, display leadership qualities, tend to be moderately affluent and enjoy fine things. They are both creative and stable.

The *pitta* pulse is known as 'the frog'. Its rate is 70–80 per minute. It is erratic.

The five types of *pitta*

There are five types of *pitta*, seated in different parts of the body: *paachaka* (the

---

CHARACTERISTICS OF THE PREDOMINANTLY *PITTA* INDIVIDUAL

- ✦ medium body, neither too light nor too heavy
- ✦ smooth skin, possibly with moles and freckles
- ✦ small eyes, often green, brown or grey
- ✦ good appetite but not prone to rapid weight gain
- ✦ medium veins, muscles and bones

- ✦ thin hair which falls out easily (males prone to baldness)
- ✦ free, often excessive perspiration
- ✦ moderate sex drive
- ✦ high intelligence, but a tendency to anger and being judgmental
- ✦ openness to new ideas
- ✦ decisiveness and leadership qualities

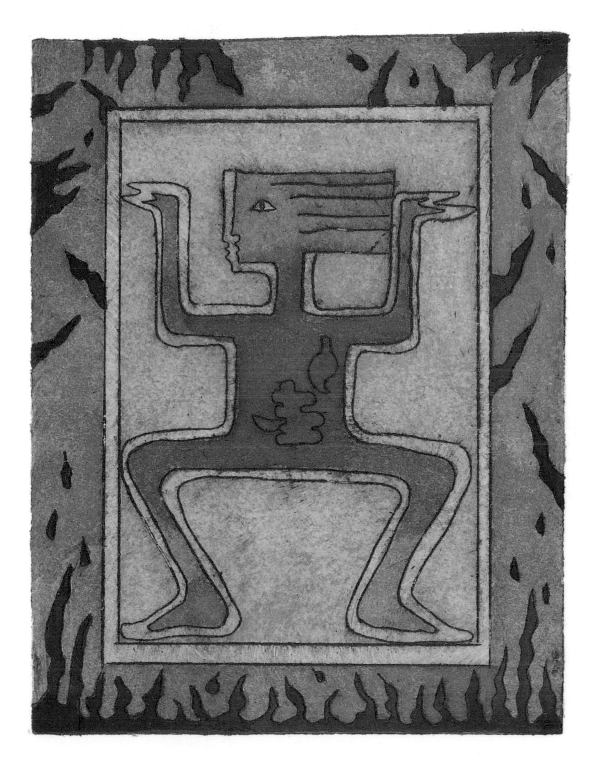

stomach), *ranjaka* (the liver), *saadhaka* (the heart), *aalochaka* (the eyes) and *bhraajaka* (the skin).

✦ **Paachaka** *pitta* resides in the stomach and is the most important *pitta* energy as it helps the other four to function properly. It influences the activities of the digestive juices (saliva, gastric juices, pancreatic juices, bile and the other enzymes which aid digestion). An imbalance leads to a malfunctioning of all five *pittas*.

✦ **Ranjana** *pitta* resides in the spleen and stomach, but mainly in the liver whose functions it influences. A healthily functioning liver is vital for the effective elimination of toxic wastes; it is the principal organ of elimination and detoxification and tends to accumulate chemical substances from Western drugs and medications. An imbalance results in a poor liver function.

✦ **Saadhaka** *pitta* resides in the heart and governs intelligence, intellect, creativity, memory, self-esteem, the ability to achieve goals, and romantic attachments. It is not yet known whether this *pitta*, which governs mental rather than physical functions, is in the heart itself or works throughout the body. An imbalance undermines the functions listed.

✦ **Aalochaka** *pitta* resides in the pupils of the eyes and influences the ability to see external objects. An imbalance results in visual disturbance.

✦ **Bhraajaka** *pitta* resides in the skin. It regulates body temperature, sweating and the secretion of sebum (which keeps the skin soft and moist). It also influences the complexion and skin colour. An imbalance results in a range of skin complaints, from psoriasis to vitiligo.

Some symptoms of a *pitta* imbalance

A *pitta* imbalance may lead to the following disorders: poor digestion, an irregular body temperature, excessive perspiration, poor eyesight, blotchy skin and other skin complaints, a tendency to heartburn, dyspepsia, irritable bowel and diarrhoea, anxiety and irritability. Most Ayurvedic practitioners consider that disorders caused by disturbed *pitta* are less serious than those due to *vata* disturbance.

KAPHA (see pages 40–41)

THE *KAPHA* ENERGY is made up of Water and Earth. It regulates water-based functions in the body and governs strength and mass. It lubricates the joints and maintains the body's immune system.

Kapha-dominant people tend to overweight; they gain weight easily and find it difficult to shed. They are inclined to be slow and ponderous. It is not unusual for those who begin life as *vata*-dominant types to become more *kapha*-dominant as they get older, accumulate material wealth and eat more than their bodies can comfortably accommodate. They often have thick, oily skin and thick, lustrous hair. They have big eyes and strong nails. They can tend to laziness and getting other people to do things for them; but they can cope with hard physical work. They sleep well and have to guard against sleeping too much.

Temperamentally, *kapha* types can seem dull, slow and resistant to change and the unfamiliar. They are inclined to conserve (energy, strength and money) rather than spend. They are tolerant, forgiving, calm and slow to anger, are often good in business and wealthy, but are slow to absorb information. They tend to be clinging and greedy in their personal relationships. They have a low sex drive and find fidelity easy. They are not prone to depression. They are more materialistic than spiritual.

The *kapha* pulse is known as 'the swan'. Its rate is 60–70 per minute. It is slow, steady, soft, broad, regular and warm

The five types of *kapha*

There are five types of *kapha*, seated in the body: *kledaka* (the stomach), *avalambaka* (the heart), *bodhaka* (the tongue), *tarpaka* (the head) and *sleshaka* (the joints).

✦ **Kledaka** *kapha* resides in the stomach. It helps to moisten food. It protects the mucous membranes in the mouth, oesophagus, stomach and intestines. An imbalance results in indigestion and abdominal cramps.

✦ **Avalambaka** *kapha* resides in the thorax. It supports the heart and the other four *kaphas* in the performance of their functions by secreting minute quantities of fluid. An imbalance results in heartburn, and weakness in the heart and lungs.

✦ **Bodhaka** *kapha* resides in the tongue and governs the ability to taste.

✦ **Tarpaka** *kapha* resides in the brain, and maintains its strength. An imbalance results in headaches, nausea, insomnia, vertigo, diarrhoea and mental disturbance.

✦ **Sleshaka** *kapha* resides in the joints and keeps them well lubricated. An imbalance results in conditions such as arthritis.

Some symptoms of a *kapha* imbalance

An imbalance of *kapha* energy may also cause the following symptoms: a thin, flabby appearance due to poor nutrition, loose joints, a weak and over-soft body, impotence, slow digestion, excess mucus and overriding feelings of jealousy, insecurity and intolerence.

CHARACTERISTICS OF THE PREDOMINANTLY *KAPHA* INDIVIDUAL

- ✦ a body prone to fat
- ✦ thick, oily hair and skin
- ✦ clear whites of the eyes
- ✦ thick, heavy eyelids,
- ✦ unprominent veins and muscles
- ✦ heavy bones

- ✦ strong-smelling body odour
- ✦ slowness, ponderousness and tendency to inactivity
- ✦ unimaginative approach to sex
- ✦ tendency to oversleep
- ✦ medium intelligence

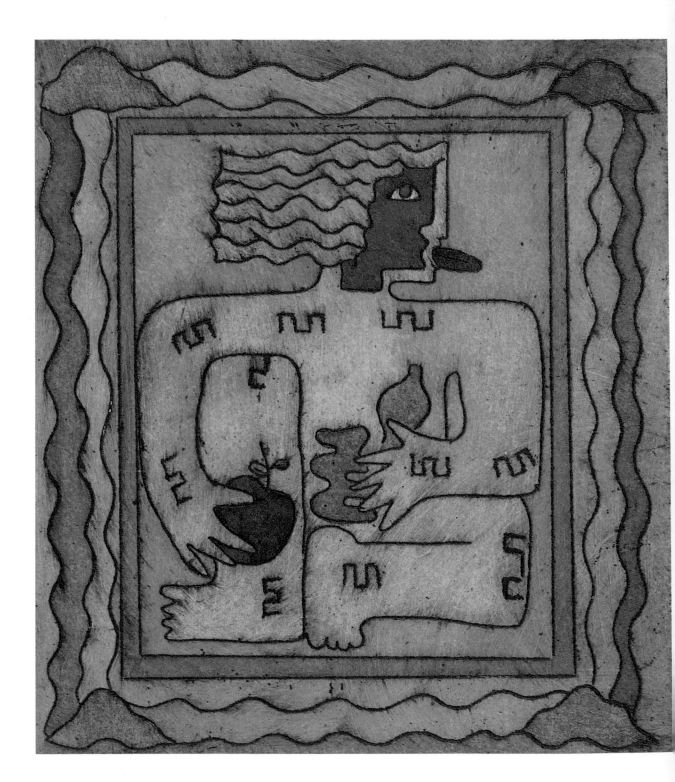

BALANCED DOSHAS

IN ADDITION TO the three main types, individuals may fall into one of several sub-groups, such as *vata-pitta, vata-kapha* or *pitta-kapha*. Those whose *doshas* are balanced are the most fortunate, but they are also the rarest. All of the energies work in perfect harmony and they are free of extremes. The aim of Ayurveda is balance, but there is only so much that any system of medicine can do. Generally, the more we live in harmony with nature, the more balanced our *doshas* become.

The Ayurvedic lifestyle (see page 70) does a lot to bring the *doshas* into balance without the need for medication or any other form of treatment. For the moment, it can be confidently stated that those who live calm, regular, well-ordered lives with a sense of purpose, who are neither anxiety-prone nor too laid-back to be bothered with anything, who eat regular meals of unprocessed foods (preferably vegetarian), who sleep regular hours and take regular exercise, and who do not take drugs or any other artificial stimulants, are most likely to achieve *dosha* balance.

THE CONSTITUTION OF THE MIND

LIKE THE BODY, the mind has its own constitution. The three types are *sattvic, rajasic* and *tamasic*.

+ ***Sattvic***, without taint or negativism, is the purest state to which the mind can aspire and is very rare. *Sattvic* people have only pure, positive thoughts both about themselves and others. They have confidence in themselves and high self-esteem, without being egotistical. They respect other people but do not let others walk all over them. They have a clear idea about what they want and take steps to achieve it. They cause no sorrow to any other living creature. They enjoy excellent physical health, favouring a pure diet free of artificial stimulants. This state does not come naturally to most people, but practising meditation and following the Buddhist noble eightfold path (see page 16) help us reach towards it. Ayurveda assists the aspiring *sattvic* with recommendations for proper diet (see page 60), meditation, exercise, thought and understanding. It is to *sattvic* that we should all aspire, even if we will never attain it.

+ The ***rajasic*** mind is passionate and angry. It can be violent, partial and subject to irrational mood swings. *Rajasic* people seek stimuli of all kinds – they enjoy rich, spicy food, eating out, the theatre, cinema, novels, alcohol, gossip and extrovert behaviour. They are restless, always on the lookout for new challenges and experiences, and are never satisfied. They are often intelligent and creative, but are never at peace, with themselves or the world.

+ The ***tamasic*** mind is low and ignorant. *Tamasic* people enjoy junky, processed foods and lack vitality and vigour. They are unintelligent, ignorant, irrational, greedy and filled with destructive thoughts and ideas. Both *rajasic* and *tamasic* attitudes are considered to be tainted and can be the cause of ill-health. *Rajasic* and *tamasic* elements in our lives removes the *sattvic* state from our reach.

THE DHAATUS

THE *SAPTA DHAATUS* are the seven essential tissues which make up the human body. Like the *doshas* (see page 25), the *dhaatus* are understood to be formed from one or more of the five elements (see page 24). Unlike the *doshas*, the *dhaatus* can be seen under a microscope and even with the naked eye.

According to Ayurvedic teaching, the *dhaatus* follow a logical sequence. *Rasa dhaatu* (plasma) is the first, and is the basis of the formation of blood (*rakta dhaatu*), which flows into the muscles (*mamsa dhaatu*). These are followed by *meda dhaatu* (fatty tissue), *asthi dhaatu* (bone and nerve tissue), *majja dhaatu* (bone marrow) and *shukra dhaatu* (reproductive tissue).

'We are what we eat'

The *dhaatus* are formed from what we eat through the process of metabolism. Ayurveda teaches that these seven essential tissues must not be lost from the system or illness will result. The metabolic process also separates nutrients from waste products and ensures that waste is eliminated from the body. Digested food then undergoes seven distinct stages through which it forms one of the seven tissues or *dhaatus*.

When the *doshas* are working in harmony, metabolism and digestion also function efficiently and the whole system will be healthy. But if any of the *doshas* is out of balance, the process will be faulty and illness will manifest itself in one or more of the tissues.

If metabolism is too rapid, too little tissue

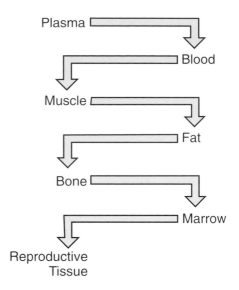

The formation of our seven body tissues.

is formed; when it is too slow, too much tissue accumulates. The whole mechanism works like a delicate instrument – if there is one flaw in the process, the whole mechanism will be out of harmony.

◆ *Rasa dhaatu* (plasma) is present in liquid form (related to the element Water). It is the fluid which, following the digestive process, contains all the nutrients which will be absorbed from the intestines. It is considered by Ayurveda to be very important and supplies nutrients to all the other *dhaatus* and, when high, promotes good skin, vigour, happiness, good memory and concentration.

◆ *Rakta dhaatu* (blood) is formed from Fire. Through the circulation of the blood, it provides oxygen to every part of the body. When the right amount of oxygen is being produced, there is a feeling of vitality, love and trust. The whole body radiates good health, and there is a reddish, plump look and feel to parts such as the lips, tongue, genitals, ears, hands and feet. If too little *Rakta dhaatu* is produced, the result is pale, dry skin, low blood pressure, and cravings for certain foods. Too much *rakta dhaatu* causes inflammation of the skin and blood vessels, and jaundice.

✦ *Mamsa dhaatu* (muscle) is related to the element of Earth. It generates muscle tissue and is responsible for the body's physical strength. When the correct amount is produced, the body is strong and healthy and there is a feeling of optimism and courage. If too little is produced, the result is weakness and wasting diseases. There is a lack of co-ordination and a feeling of extreme tiredness. Overproduction of this *dhaatu* can cause swellings and tumours, obesity, irritability and aggression and can cause fibroids in women which may result in miscarriage and infertility.

✦ *Meda dhaatu* (fatty tissue) is related to the elements of Water and Earth. It is responsible for lubricating muscles, ligaments and joints. The correct quantity of this tissue enables muscles and joints to work smoothly and efficiently, and generates a feeling of being loved and cared for. (Some Ayurvedic practitioners believe that a powerful cause of excessive weight gain is a feeling of being unloved and not cared for sufficiently. Subconsciously, the person who is overweight believes that layers of fat compensate for a feeling of inner emptiness, making it even more difficult for a chronically overweight person to lose excess fat.)

✦ *Asthi dhaatu* (bone and nerve tissue) is formed from Air and Earth. It provides the structure for all other body tissues. It generates feelings of security, stability and endurance. It is believed that *vata* energy resides in bone tissue.

✦ *Majja dhaatu* (marrow) is formed from Water. The principal function of bone marrow is to fill hollow spaces, such as the interior of bones, with tissue which produces blood cells. It also provides essential fluid to moisten eyes, skin and the stools. When the right amount is produced, there is a feeling of fulfilment.

✦ *Shukra dhaatu* (reproductive tissue). The principal function of this tissue is the creation of new life. *Shukra* means 'semen', but by modern extension (as attitudes have evolved, and the emphasis on male dominance has diminished) it is taken also to refer to female reproductive tissue. The waste product of *shukra dhaatu* is smegma.

When *shukra dhaatu* is not produced effectively, there can be difficulties with potency and ejaculation, a loss of sex drive, a weakened immune system and back pain.

Overproduction of *shukra dhaatu* can lead to sexual hyperactivity, excessive discharge, irascibility and an enlarged prostate in men.

This tissue also controls the effectiveness of the body's immune system which protects against chronic infections. Ayurvedic practitioners believe that excessive sexual activity will lead to exaustion and produce low quality sperm which may create a weak baby.

WHAT TYPE ARE YOU?

Here is a checklist of the main characteristics of each main dosha type from which it is possible to establish your dominant dosha. The most common disorders to which each type is particularly prone are also listed together with recommendations of diet, exercise, lifestyle and Ayurvedic treatments to counter the effects of excessive dosha.

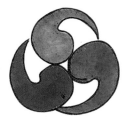

Prakruti (the physical constitution)

It is important for doctor and patient to understand the concept and function of the doshas, so that no treatment is offered which works against a predominant dosha (see page 26). The individual constitution is evaluated to form the basis of the Ayurvedic diagnosis. A person should maintain their original dosha levels throughout their life. If these change for any reason, it leads to abnormal dosha levels, producing a state of imbalance known as vikruti.

The ages of **dosha** dominance
As a general rule:
✦ kapha-related problems are common from birth to the age of twenty
✦ pitta-related problems are common between the ages of twenty and fifty years.
✦ vata-related problems are common after the age of fifty years

Characteristics of *vata*

A variable appetite; little perspiration; frequent but sparse urine; hard, dark stools and a tendency to constipation; a highly original and creative mind; a poor to average memory; indecisiveness; rapid speech; wastefulness with money; nervousness and shyness; a tendency to anxiety and depression; a high sex drive (or none at all); a love of travel; high mobility; a dislike of cold weather and strong winds.

Health problems associated with *vata*

Heart problems; disorders of the nervous system; anxiety; tension; hypertension; depression; migraine; irritable bowel syndrome.

How to live with *vata*

✦ avoid eating foods high in vata (see chart on page 66–7) and eat pitta- and kapha-increasing food
✦ eat moderately warm food (warm milk is a beneficial drink); avoid cold or frozen food
✦ choose sweet, acid and salty foods; avoid hot and spicy food, and reduce your intake of nuts and seeds
✦ massage with vata oils (see page 47)
✦ use steam baths with vata oil applications
✦ with the supervision of an Ayurvedic practitioner, cleanse the digestive system and body with oils, salty liquids, Ayurvedic preparations and panchakarma methods regularly
✦ avoid excessive physical activities
✦ make sure to get plenty of rest and listen to relaxing music
✦ meditate every day

Characteristics of *pitta*

A strong appetite; a tendency to sweat; frequent need to urinate; loose stools and a tendency to diarrhoea; loud speech; an interest in technical and scientific matters; care with money; a tendency to jealousy, ambition and egotism; a passionate and dominating sex drive; a love of sport; an interest in politics; a love of luxury; a dislike of heat.

Health problems associated with pitta

Ulcers; digestive problems; gall bladder and liver problems; skin complaints; headaches.

How to live with *pitta*

◆ avoid eating foods high in pitta (see the chart on page 66–7)
◆ eat vata and kapha increasing food
◆ eat cooling food (drinking cold water, eating ghee and taking suitable oils are beneficial)
◆ eat a high proportion of raw foods, i.e. salads, fruits and vegetables; avoid pickles, fizzy and acidic drinks and reduce your intake of fruit juice
◆ avoid excess alcohol, salt, tea and coffee
◆ choose sweet, bitter and astringent food
◆ take yoghurt after meals
◆ drink plenty of liquids
◆ try to maintain a cool environment – bathe in cool water
◆ swimming in cold water,
taking walks in moonlight and living near water are all beneficial activities for pitta types
◆ massage the body with pitta oils
◆ do not expose the body to too much sun

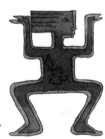

Characteristics of *kapha*

A moderate to sluggish appetite; heavy sweating; profuse but infrequent urination; large, soft stools; melodious speech; a businesslike approach; a good memory; careful decision making; thrift and care with money; a tendency to save and conserve; monogamy; lethargy and passivity; a love of peace and quiet and familiar places; a love of good food; a dislike of cold, damp conditions.

Health problems associated with *kapha*

Hypertension; heart disease; circulatory disorders; diabetes; gall bladder problems; eczema; asthma; sinusitis; bronchitis.

How to live with *kapha*

◆ avoid eating foods high in kapha (see the chart on page 66–7)
◆ eat hot and spicy food
◆ avoid cold and raw food
◆ do not snack between meals
◆ avoid fatty and fried food, meat and meat products and excess oil
◆ avoid alcohol consumption and control addictions to sweet food
◆ choose heating, bitter, pungent and astringent food
◆ take walks after meals
◆ avoid a cold environment
◆ take warm baths and wear warm clothing
◆ avoid excess sleep
◆ cleanse the body with panchakarma therapy regularly
◆ massage the body with kapha oils
◆ engage in daily physical activity

OJA

A SECONDARY PRODUCT of *shukra dhaatu* is a substance with no physical form, but which is often referred to as the 'eighth body tissue'. It is called *oja* and in Ayurvedic teaching is regarded as life's energy. It is the ultimate vital energy pervading the system and is said to reside throughout the body. Some Ayurvedic practitioners believe that it particularly pervades the lymphatic system and therefore influences immunity. It supports all of the body's functions which depend for their effectiveness upon regular meditation and following a healthy lifestyle, such as moderate habits, good food and regular sleep. Eating unsuitable food and indulging in sexual overactivity decreases *oja*.

There are many diseases and conditions for which orthodox medicine can find no proven cause and for which there is no cure. Ayurvedic practitioners believe that reduced levels of *oja* allow infections (both viral and bacterial) to settle in the body. *Oja* is transformed into *theja*, which reflects personal levels of energy, a personal 'aura' of spiritual development. *Oja* and *theja* could be described as a type of stamina. People with less of it generally tend to have a weakened system.

A predetermined order

As already suggested, the *dhaatus,* or tissues, are formed in a predetermined order of precedence. Plasma becomes blood, blood becomes muscle, muscle becomes fat, fat becomes bone, bone becomes marrow, and marrow becomes reproductive tissue. The last is the tissue with the highest potential – to create new life and perpetuate the species. As all body tissues are formed through the ingestion of food, it is essential to take in only high-quality, nutritious foods. Rubbishy foods create unhealthy body tissue and a correspondingly unhealthy mental condition.

The importance of diet is discussed in detail on pages 56–69.

THE MALAS

THE EFFICIENT ELIMINATION of waste products (*malas)* is as important as eating and drinking the right nutrients. Ayurveda teaches that there are three main waste products of the body's metabolic process: faeces (*shakrit* or *pureesha*), urine (*mootra*) and sweat (*sweda*).

Ama

A further type of digestive waste (*ama*) is an accumulation of toxic materials and a result of an unhealthy diet and lifestyle and the ingestion of toxins. Strictly speaking, it should not be present in the body, which has no mechanism for its elimination and it is, therefore, not considered one of the *malas*. Accumulation of *ama* always leads to disease.

If elimination is faulty, any of the *malas* can cause disease. Serious illness can result if waste products are not eliminated efficiently and are re-absorbed by the body. An Ayurvedic doctor needs information about a patient's eliminative processes, and will ask many questions to facilitate accurate diagnosis and advise you upon the appropriate treatment for your *dosha* type and your condition.

✦ **Shakrit or pureesha** (faeces). When the body's digestive processes are functioning normally, about a litre of fluid reaches the colon every day. This fluid, which consists of fibre, unwanted food debris and residue, is converted into solid faeces. The Earth element converts food residue into a form suitable for elimination by the colon. This process is controlled by the *vata dosha* and is essential for the healthy functioning of all the organs of the body. If waste matter is not eliminated, and is absorbed back into the system, the resulting disorders can include osteoarthritis, bronchitis, asthma, low back pain and headaches.

✦ **Mootra** (urine). The formation of urine begins in the kidneys. The urinary system acts to remove waste salts and, when these are eliminated efficiently, the body will be in good health. Orthodox medicine now recognises, as Ayurveda has known for centuries, that urine tests reveal a lot about a patient's general state of health and *dosha* status. Inefficient elimination of urine can result in the following symptoms: abdominal distention, a burning sensation when urinating, and inflammation and infections of the bladder and kidneys.

✦ **Sweda** (sweat). Sweat is formed principally from water and originates in the body's fatty tissue. Perspiration is essential for detoxification and maintaining even body temperature and removing watery waste. An inability to sweat causes dry skin and burning sensations and an important part of Ayurvedic therapy is the inducement of sweating. Too much sweating, on the other hand, can cause fungal infections, such as ringworm, and unpleasant body odour results from the action of accumulated bacteria.

Other excretions and waste products, such as hair, nails, ear wax and secretions from the eyes and genitals do not in themselves normally cause disease.

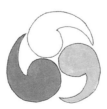

The Unique
Individual

For Ayurvedic treatment to be effective, it is essential that doctor and patient recognise the latter's constitutional type. Everybody's constitution has three principal elements – the *doshas*, genetic inheritance and *karma*. The *doshas* are the prevailing energies which determine basic body type (see page 25); from parents, grandparents and all our ancestors we inherit characteristics and, in some cases, a predisposition to certain diseases and conditions, and, through *karma*, we bring aspects and propensities to this existence from previous incarnations. The three factors interact to give every individual a unique constitution, established by the time we are born and unchangeable. With the passage of time, however, the constitution can be affected by factors such as diet, habits, lifestyle, the environment, exercise (or lack of it), work, hormonal changes and stress.

THE MARMAS

AS HAS ALREADY been suggested, Ayurveda regards every person as unique with an individual physical and psychological constitution, determined by genetic inheritance, *dosha* influence and *karma.* Although many changes occur in our bodies and our minds as we go through life, we remain essentially the same person we were at birth unless we impose a *doshic* imbalance upon ourselves with an unhealthy lifestyle.

Ayurveda identifies a factor which connects the different stages of our lives and maintains our individual identity. It is called *smirti,* which can translate as 'memory', which permeates evey cell in our body. Ayurveda also teaches us that to be healthy in this life, we must allow vital energy, or *prana,* to flow unimpeded through them. If our posture is poor, or we indulge in thoughts and attitudes which cramp our style and make us resentful and angry, that energy is blocked. Our bodies and minds cannot then function harmoniously, making it impossible for us to live to our full potential.

The matrix of energy points

There are a large number of energy points (107 in all) in the body which stimulate some of its functions and maintain health by keeping them in equilibrium. Although these points (known as *marmas* or *marmasthans*) cannot be located using scientific instruments, there is considered to be sufficient evidence that whenever one or other of them malfunctions or becomes blocked, illness sets in. Most are in vital areas such as tendons, major arteries and veins, and the principal joints.

Ayurvedic texts suggest that the *marma* points are parts of the body where two or more important systems meet, such as nerves and blood vessels, bones and nerves, or muscles, ligaments and joints. A *marma* point is the site of concentrated energy, and damage to any of these points can lead to serious illness.

There are three main *marma* centres: the head; the heart and the bladder. Violent injury to any of these *marma* centres can result in death.

The legacy of past lives

Ayurveda also teaches that the *marma* points can be used to manipulate the forces of *vata, pitta* and *kapha* (see page 25). In some people, the flow of *prana* through the points may be blocked by 'memories' brought from previous lives. While these memories may not be conscious, they and any traumas associated with them nevertheless can have a profound effect upon a person. A new-born child's behaviour is influenced by what has happened to it in past lives, but as its life proceeds, those memories are eclipsed by new experiences.

Ayurveda is not alone in its belief in past lives. Hypnotic regression has appeared to demonstrate that people have lived before and their memories of previous existences can be unlocked and explored. Differences among those who concede the possibility of our having lived before usually focus on interpretation with a gamut of explanations ranging from reincarnation to folk memory. And there are, of course, many who refuse to countenance the possibility at all and prefer a scientific explanation of characteristics such as that offered by genetics. Inevitably it comes down to a question of belief and personal experience. It is a major plank of Ayurveda. Unless one believes in reincarnation and *karma,* the world appears chaotic, meaningless, anarchic and unjust. Followers of Ayurveda do not accept this view of the world, but believe that all things work according to ordered principles.

When a disease occurs for no obvious reason, as is often the case with children, Ayurveda believes that a predisposition to the condition has been brought by the sufferer from a previous life. Our *marma* points are blocked at birth as they are self-regulating mechanisms. Similarly, phobias may relate to experiences in previous lives. A fear of spiders or flying may be caused by 'memories' brought to this life from earlier lives. The task of the Ayurvedic physician is to apply specific treatment to the *marma* points to unblock the energy and allow *prana* to flow freely and eliminate disease.

Marma therapy

Treatment applied to the *marma* points can influence bodily functions in much the same way acupuncture is believed to. In fact, it is thought that in ancient times, some parts of Ayurvedic texts, which describe *marma* therapy in detail, were taken to China and the theory was developed into acupuncture. In more recent times massage of or applying pressure to the *marma* points has been shown to produce beneficial effects. Conditions successfully treated this way include anxiety and tension; arthritis; chronic fatigue; frozen shoulder; immune disorders; irritable bowel syndrome; lack of vitality; migraine; neuromuscular lesions; skin complaints and tennis elbow, as well as specific problems associated with particular *marma* points – for example, a problem with a *marma* point in the knee can cause constipation.

Marma puncture

Marma puncture is the Ayurvedic equivalent of acupuncture and is effective in treating conditions which do not respond to orthodox medicine. Applying gentle pressure to the correct points can bring relief. The treatment is also carried out using appropriate massage techniques and oils, which vary according to which *dosha* is dominant. One of the most popular, *narayana* oil, is derived from a mixture of herbs which are highly effective in the treatment of *vata*-oriented problems. It is applied as a hot poultice and accompanies a kneading form of massage. Oils recommended for the different *dosha* types are:

+ *Vata* – calming oils (sesame, olive, almond, amla, bala, wheat germ, castor).
+ *Pitta* – cooling oils (coconut, sandal wood, pumpkin seed, almond, sunflower).
+ *Kapha* – burning oils (sesame, safflower, mustard, corn).

These recommendations reflect yet again the importance of treating individuals in accordance with their *dosha* types.

There is a wide range of multi-herbal preparations available which your Ayurvedic practitioner may recommend (see page 122).

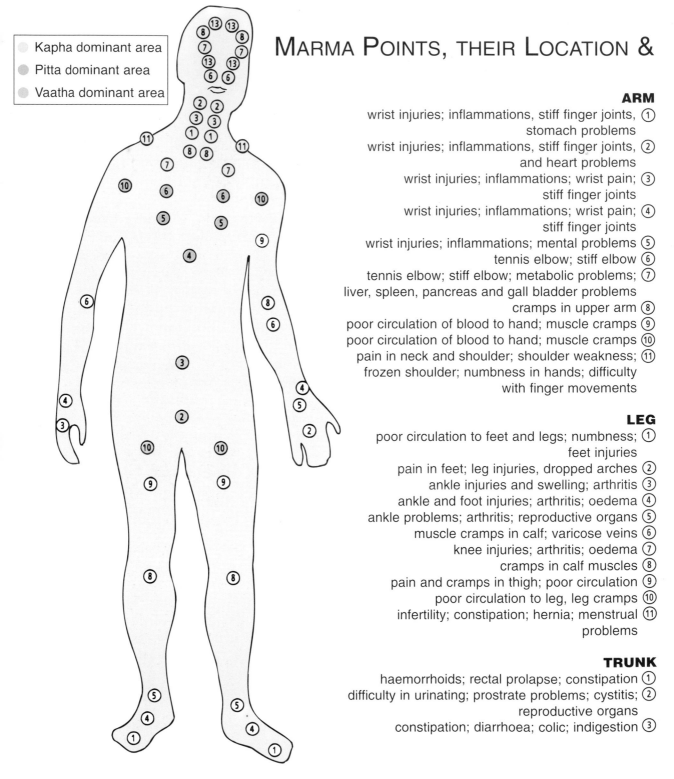

Kapha dominant area

Pitta dominant area

Vaatha dominant area

MARMA POINTS, THEIR LOCATION &

ARM

wrist injuries; inflammations, stiff finger joints, ①
stomach problems

wrist injuries; inflammations, stiff finger joints, ②
and heart problems

wrist injuries; inflammations; wrist pain; ③
stiff finger joints

wrist injuries; inflammations; wrist pain; ④
stiff finger joints

wrist injuries; inflammations; mental problems ⑤

tennis elbow; stiff elbow ⑥

tennis elbow; stiff elbow; metabolic problems; ⑦
liver, spleen, pancreas and gall bladder problems

cramps in upper arm ⑧

poor circulation of blood to hand; muscle cramps ⑨

poor circulation of blood to hand; muscle cramps ⑩

pain in neck and shoulder; shoulder weakness; ⑪
frozen shoulder; numbness in hands; difficulty
with finger movements

LEG

poor circulation to feet and legs; numbness; ①
feet injuries

pain in feet; leg injuries, dropped arches ②

ankle injuries and swelling; arthritis ③

ankle and foot injuries; arthritis; oedema ④

ankle problems; arthritis; reproductive organs ⑤

muscle cramps in calf; varicose veins ⑥

knee injuries; arthritis; oedema ⑦

cramps in calf muscles ⑧

pain and cramps in thigh; poor circulation ⑨

poor circulation to leg, leg cramps ⑩

infertility; constipation; hernia; menstrual ⑪
problems

TRUNK

haemorrhoids; rectal prolapse; constipation ①

difficulty in urinating; prostrate problems; cystitis; ②
reproductive organs

constipation; diarrhoea; colic; indigestion ③

RELATED PHYSICAL SYMPTOMS

TRUNK

④ heart diseases; high blood pressure; low blood pressure; poor circulation

⑤ mastitis; engorged breasts; tender breasts; lack of milk production

⑥ mastitis; engorged breasts with inflammation

⑦ shoulder cramps; injuries; breathing difficulty

⑧ bronchitis; asthma; difficulty in breathing; panic attacks

BACK

① sciatica; pain in leg; muscle cramps in leg; weakness in leg; paralysis; arthritis in hip

② arthritis in hip; injury to hip

③ low back pain; stiff back

④ sacro-iliac joint problems; lumbar back pain; sciatica; reproductive organs

⑤ stiff neck; neck injuries; headaches

⑥ shoulder pain; injury; muscle cramps in shoulder blade

⑦ weakness in hands; paralysis; numbness

NECK

① headache; speech difficulty; paralysis

② stammering; paralysis; sore throat; cough; thyroid problems

③ stiff neck; speech problems; throat infections; thyroid problems

④ stiff neck; headache; neck injury; stammering

⑤ dizziness; vertigo; deafness; inflammation in ear

⑥ loss of sense of smell; catarrh; rhinitis; nasal polyp

⑦ trigeminal neuralgia; headache; facial paralysis

⑧ migraine; vertigo; loss of hearing; loss of memory

⑨ migraine; vertigo; loss of memory

⑩ migraine, headaches; vertigo

⑪ loss of smell; catarrh; pituitary problems

⑫ headaches; convulsions; epilepsy; memory loss

⑬ sinusitis; frontal headache

⑭ headache; migraine; memory loss; paralysis; lack of energy

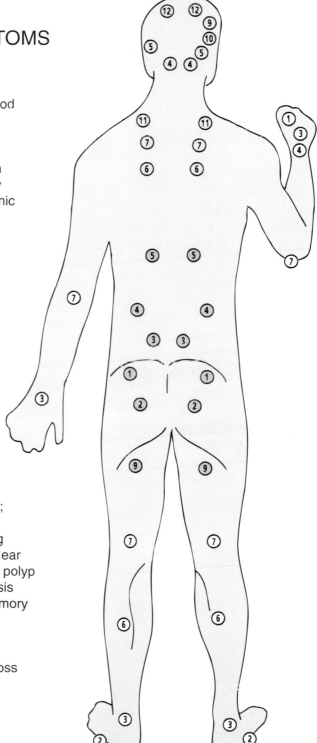

CASE STUDIES

✦ Migraine

Margaret (45) had suffered from migraine for fifteen years and it was getting worse. Although taking strong painkillers prescribed by her doctor, she was having a severe attack almost once a week. Reluctant to be sentenced to a life on painkillers, she turned to Ayurveda. Much of Margaret's liver function had been destroyed by her prescription drugs. She is a predominantly *vata* type (migraine is associated with a disturbance of *vata* energy) and was thin, restless and always on the go. After examining her, the Ayurvedic doctor prescribed *panchakarma* therapy (Margaret had experienced colonic irrigation, so did not find the treatment unnerving), which was followed by oral herbal preparations and *marma puncture*. She was asked to return every two weeks. Some modifications were suggested to Margaret's diet. Wheat and wheat products, tomatoes, strawberries, aubergines, pickled food and acidic fruit juices were excluded, as was all alcohol. As a journalist, Margaret had many working lunches and, although she found it difficult to stick to the diet, she persevered. After three months, she suffered only one mild attack and she now seems to be cured. Migraine is notoriously difficult to treat successfully. Most doctors aim for a 75% success rate; 100% is extremely rare.

Julie (36), a solicitor practising in a busy inner-city office, had suffered from migraine for five years. She had tried many treatments without signs of improvement and was becoming desperate. Her condition became so bad that she was afflicted as many as two attacks every week.

When she came to see me I prescribed a course of detoxification, an Ayurvedic diet and a course of *marma puncture*. After six months' treatment she had only had one attack. Her life was improved immeasurably.

✦ Chronic Mastitis

Linda (38), married with two children, had suffered from mastitis for two years. Her GP had tried all the treatments available to him with no success. A test for hormonal imbalance had not found anything amiss. Linda suffered constantly from swollen and tender breasts and continuous discharge from the nipples. When she came to my clinic she was identified as a *vata-pitta* type and was treated with a complete detoxification programme, including a cleansing diet combined with herbal preparations and *marma puncture*. Within four weeks the health of her breasts was restored.

✦ Eczema

Adrian (36), a businessman living in London, had suffered from eczema for fifteen years. His condition tended to worsen during the summer months and at times of stress. Adrian had tried steroidal creams and the oral medications prescribed by his GP but they only provided temporary relief. There seemed to be no cure. He then turned to Ayurveda and

CASE STUDIES

was diagnosed as a *vata-pitta* type (a very warm body with dry skin). His treatment consisted of a new diet, exercises, oral medication, *panchakarma* and regular *marma puncture* over a three-month period. His eczema gradually disappeared and now he visits the clinic once a month.

✦ Hypertension

Harold (67) is an accountant with a very stressful lifestyle but no history of hypertension in the family. Harold had suffered for twenty years from it and had been taking diuretics and beta-blockers prescribed by his GP for his high blood pressure. He did not want to take these pills for the rest of his life but he realised that his life was so busy that he could not afford not to function.

He approached Ayurveda (tentatively at first, because he had mixed views about embracing a complementary therapy which initially seemed rather alien to him) while continuing to follow the recommendations of his GP. His lifestyle up until that point proved to be the main cause of his problems. His programme of Ayurvedic treatments included a new diet, oral medications, *panchakarma* which included steam bath treatment (*sweda karma*), yoga, meditation and *marma puncture*.

The *marma puncture* was used to relieve his stress and tension, and very often he would fall into a deep sleep during the therapy session. When his blood pressure had remained stable for two months his GP agreed that he could gradually withdraw from

the drugs. From then on Harold simply carried on his diet, meditation and exercise plan and now he only visits the clinic once a month for *marma puncture*.

Carin (47) came to see me five years ago after her GP had diagnosed high blood pressure. He had prescribed beta-blockers and diuretics. But the beta-blockers did not agree with her and she started to suffer from undesirable side-effects. She decided that her life would be made miserable if she had to spend the rest of her years taking such drugs.

Over a period of six months I treated her with *marma puncture*, Ayurveda herbal preparations and *panchakarma*. After three months' treatment she withdrew from her GP's medication under supervision. Very soon she was maintaining a normal pressure without the Ayurvedic preparations because she was responding to *marma puncture* so well. She now visits the clinic once a month for *marma puncture* and once every three months for *panchakarma* therapy.

✦ Postnatal depression

This condition is quite common in the West. Orthodox practitioners believe that it is caused by a lack of oestrogen in the system after birth.

Ayurvedic cleansing treatments, supported with practices such as meditation and yoga, have been very successful in treating postnatal depression and many mothers find themselves cured after a few short sessions.

THE CHAKRAS

THE CONCEPT OF the *chakras* is likely to be familiar to anyone who has studied yoga. Charts of the *chakras* can be seen in any yoga centre and in books about yoga. There are seven and they are perceived to be circles located along the midline of the body in line with the spinal chord (except for the lowest which is located in the genital area and the highest which is located above the head). According to ancient teaching, the aim should be to enable a type of energy called *kundalini* to move from the lowest *chakra* to the highest to promote spirituality and divine knowledge.

◆ *Muladhara* is the lowest *chakra*, located between the genitals and the anus.

◆ *Svadisthana* is the second *chakra* and lies in the sacral region.

◆ *Manipura*, the third *chakra*, is located in the solar plexus.

◆ *Anahata* is the fourth *chakra* and is located in the spine at heart level.

◆ *Vishuddha*, the fifth *chakra*, is situated in the neck.

◆ *Ajna* is located in the forehead between the eyebrows (at the point where Indian women wear a red dot and where the 'third eye' was considered to be).

◆ *Sahasrara*, the seventh *chakra*, is located just above the head and does not, therefore, have a 'physical' position.

Because the *chakras* have no physical manifestation and cannot be located using any scientific instrument, they have tended to be viewed with extreme scepticism by Western doctors, a distinction they share with the notion of meridians, and energy points in acupuncture. Instead, they are believed to have been sensed intuitively by many people over many centuries. It is certainly true that people in yoga positions and in deep meditation have experienced the sensation of a surge of energy rising from the base of the spine and emerging through the top of the head. Some people have said they have seen points of blue light when their *kundalini* energy has risen from the lowest *chakra* to the highest and they have also experienced a profound feeling of happiness.

Some believe that *kundalini* energy manifests itself when sexual desire is sublimated and turned into its spiritual, non-physical expression. Those who have achieved bliss through meditation have described it as more ecstatic than the most satisfying sexual experience. Both yoga and meditation techniques are designed to activate *kundalini* energy and bring it into balance. Allowing powerful energy centres to remain clear and unblocked is a highly effective form of preventive medicine. This can be achieved with meditation, yoga, *chakra* massage or *marma puncture* (see the case studies on pages 50–1).

The chakras, *centres of energy located along* ▶ *the midline of the body, are related to the three main* marma *centres which receive energy generated by the* chakras *and distribute it to the other 107* marma *points in the body.*

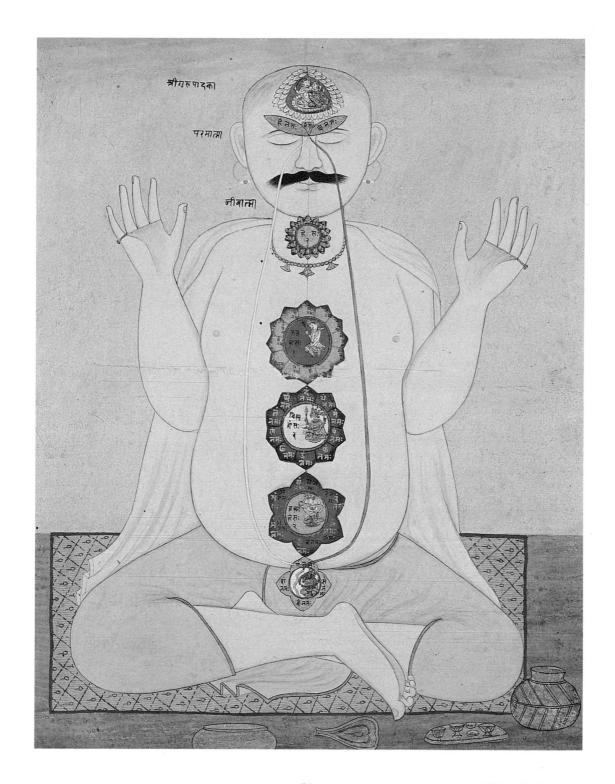

The *chakras* are believed to correspond to the *marmas* in the body, and it is believed that the *chakras* generate energy and transmit it directly to their corresponding *marma* centres, which in turn distribute energy to the 107 *marma* points in the body (see pages 48–9).

The results of blocked *chakras*

According to Ayurveda, the following disorders result when any of the *chakras* is blocked.

✦ *Prana vayu*: breathlessness, panic attacks, depression, insomnia, memory loss, physical debility, lack of energy, loss of concentration, mood swings, brain disorders.

✦ *Udana vayu*: speech difficulties, breathing problems, panic attacks, hyperventilation, asthma, bronchitis, laryngitis, thyroid malfunction.

✦ *Samana vayu*: acidity, indigestion, peptic ulcers, lack of appetite (or the opposite, compulsive eating), bowel malfunction, gall bladder and kidney problems.

✦ *Vyaana vayu*: high or low blood pressure, heart disease, circulation problems, cold hands and feet, varicose veins, lymphatic obstructions.

✦ *Apaana vayu*: haemorrhoids, constipation, rectal or uterine prolapse, hernia, sterility, impotence, gynaecological disorders, miscarriage, prostate problems, bladder complaints.

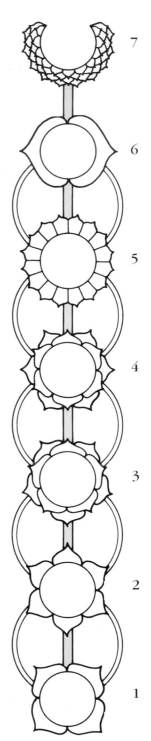

The Chakras

Leading Western scientists are now finding that the *chakras* correspond to the pathways of the brain and the immune system. In Ayurvedic belief each *chakra* corresponds to a colour and is represented by a number of petals. When practising yoga and meditation, the flow of *kundalini* (energy) passes up the line of the spine. The goal is to attain the highest level or *sahasrara* and communicate with cosmic energies.

7 **Sahasrara,** at the crown of the head, has one thousand petals and is the level of superconsciousness or *samadhi*, a level beyond time, space and consciousness.

6 **Ajna** is represented as a snow-white, two-petalled *chakra*. It is the seat of the mind and its *mantra* is OM.

5 **Vishuddha**, is represented as a blue, sixteen-petalled *chakra*. Its element is Ether and its mantra is HAM.

4 **Anahata** is represented as a grey, twelve-petalled *chakra*. Its element is Air and its mantra is YAM.

3 **Manipura** is represented as a red, ten-petalled *chakra*. Its element is Fire. Its mantra is RAM.

2 **Svadisthana** is represented as a white, six-petalled *chakra*. Its element is Water and its mantra is VAM.

1 **Muladhara** is represented as a yellow, four-petalled *chakra*. Its element is Earth and its mantra is LAM.

CASE STUDY

Chakra *massage can relieve blocked channels of energy and your Ayurvedic practitioner may recommend it to treat your condition.*

✦ **I B S** (irritable bowel syndrome)
John (44), a publisher, had suffered from this distressing condition for many years. His very busy life is made quite stressful because of the demands of his job and his family. Stress aggravates this condition. He found it very hard to cope and eventually decided that he had to find a cure.

When John visited the Ayurveda clinic he was identified as having very high levels of *vata* and low *pitta* and *kapha*. According to Ayurveda, IBS symptoms are the result of congested *prana vata* and *apana vata*, causing irregular bowel movements and low digestive fire (*agni*).

John's *chakras* needed clearing, mainly in the head and the solar plexus. He was given a full massage with great attention to the main *chakras* using *maha narayana* oil which has a *vata*-subduing and toning effect. John was also advised to take regular Ayurvedic medication and to practise yoga. It was also recommended that he modify his lifestyle to reduce the stress in his life.

John found the treatment extremely relaxing and enjoyable. He was pleasantly surprised to find just how practical and straight-forward the adjustments to his lifestyle were to make (based as they are on common sense). His condition improved markedly and within five months he was fully recovered. He has not suffered since that time.

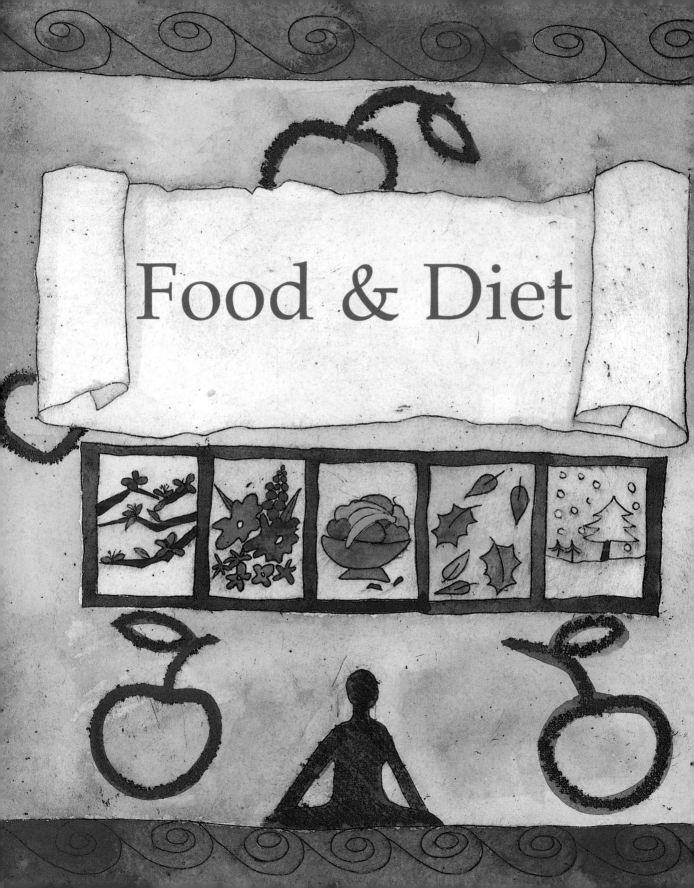

Food & Diet

In some Western countries, there has been a tradition of regarding food merely as 'fuel' for the body, not to be particularly enjoyed but to be got out of the way as quickly as possible so that everyone can get on with something more important. Opinions are divided about the merits of gathering the family together for at least one meal each day. And the development of patent drugs has tended to eclipse the view that some foodstuffs have beneficial, therapeutic and even medicinal properties. Attitudes to food vary from culture to culture. Traditionally, Indian people have always recognised both the nutritional value and the health aspects of different foods and these play an important part in simple household medicine. The idea that you should eat more of or avoid certain foodstuffs according to your individual constitution is a relatively recent idea among Western dieticians.

AYURVEDA RECOMMENDS WHICH foods to eat and which to avoid, and there are even recommendations about which food combinations are potentially harmful – a relatively recent concept in Western nutritional therapy.

Ayurveda places great importance on correct eating and drinking to promote good health and to prevent disease. It teaches that a diet of pure, unadulterated, unprocessed foods helps the body to remain healthy and avoids the accumulation of toxins.

Equally important is the recognition that different types of people need different kinds of food to maximise health. One reason why many slimming diets fail is that they take no account of different body types, metabolic rates and temperaments. The manufacturers of slimming aids appear to believe that everyone is the same, with identical body functions.

Ayurveda can help to find the most suitable diet for each individual. Its general advice is that food should be as natural as possible; avoid snacking between meals, and do not eat a large meal just before bed.

Ayurveda divides all food into two types – heavy and light. Heavy foods are those which are difficult to digest (e.g., carbohydrates, lentils, potatoes and rice); light foods (such as cooked vegetables) are easily digested. A properly balanced meal should consist of three parts 'heavy' food to one part 'light'. But there is, of course, more to it than that.

Shad rasa – the six tastes

Ayurveda divides flavours into six general groups - sweet, acidic, salty, pungent, bitter and astringent (see also page 108).

GENERAL GUIDELINES

Food should be enjoyed as well as providing nutrition. Ayurvedic practitioners recommend a list of dos and don'ts to maximise digestive processes and promote good health.

DO:

✦ Eat to satisfy your own requirements, nobody else's
✦ Choose the quality and quantity of food which you know suits you
✦ Keep tableware and the eating environment spotlessly clean
✦ Eat at a moderate pace – neither too quickly nor too slowly
✦ Pay full attention to the food you eat
✦ Eat food at the right temperature – neither too hot nor too cold
✦ Eat foods which are compatible with one another, otherwise small amounts may be left undigested and accumulate as *ama* (see page 42). This notion finds an echo in the popular Hay Diet and others which are based on food combinations. For example, proteins and carbohydrates should not be eaten together as different gastric juices are needed to digest them properly.

DON'T:

✦ Talk while eating – it is impossible to concentrate on both
✦ Laugh while eating – vibrations in the stomach impede digestion
✦ Eat until the previous meal has been fully digested – on average five hours
✦ Snack between meals

THE SEASONS

APPETITE AND DIGESTIVE function vary according to season, with the variations less obviously marked in parts of the world where seasonal climatic variation is less marked. A diet which is appropriate in summer, for example, would be unsuitable in winter. The wrong diet tends to unbalance the *doshas* and increase the risk of illness. The body adapts and its needs vary at different times of the year. (Ayurveda teaches that someone born in one type of climate should not go to live in an area which has a radically different climate.) Seasonal recommendations include the following:

Spring

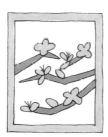

+ As digestive function is reduced and *kapha* is reduced, food with high acid content should be reduced as it can cause stomach ulcers
+ Sweet foods should be avoided as much as possible because the body finds it difficult to burn up calories
+ Additionally, sleep should be avoided during the day. Suitable exercise should be taken. Warm baths should be taken.

Summer

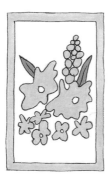

+ Cold, sweet, soft foods (such as ice cream) cool the body
+ Acid and bitter food, and heat-producing food should be avoided
+ Alcohol should be avoided, or at least diluted

+ The living environment should be kept as cool as possible
+ Additionally, exposure to moonlight is beneficial (the ancients believed that walking in the moonlight has a calming effect). Massage is beneficial as it reconditions and prepares the body for the next season. Sex should be avoided to conserve energy.

Autumn

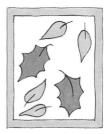

+ *Pitta* increases
+ Cold, light foods are appropriate
+ Additionally, walking in the light of the moon is recommended.

Winter

+ Digestive function increases, therefore heavier foods are digested more easily. Light foods are not suitable and, because the digestive system is more active, would increase *kapha*
+ *Vata* energy is increased
+ Salty and acidic foods can be eaten
+ Warm, comforting foods, such as milk, meat, honey, oil and rice can be enjoyed
+ Metabolism is speeded up
+ In addition, Ayurvedic herbal oils should be applied to create and conserve body heat. Suitable oils should be applied to the scalp. Warm clothing should be worn.

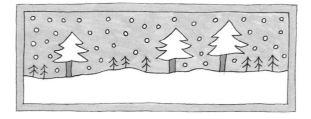

PARDON ME!

IT WAS SUGGESTED earlier that suppressing the emotions can lead to illness. Similarly, bodily functions should be allowed to happen naturally as suppressing them may also damage the system. Some account has to be taken of social convention, but the following functions should be allowed their proper role whenever possible at the proper time and in the proper place: urination; defecation (especially important); ejaculation (of sperm); breaking wind; vomiting; sneezing; yawning; satisfying hunger; slaking thirst; shedding tears; sleep; heavy breathing after exercise.

ALCOHOL

THE CONSUMPTION OF alcohol is not normally recommended as alcohol is an anti-nutrient (that is, it acts to diminish the nutritional content of food and other drinks). It is recognised, however, that a moderate intake of alcohol can have a calming effect, lead to a feeling of well-being, stimulate the digestive process and suppress the appetite. Occasionally, therefore, it may be recommended for people with an excessive appetite, those bearing great sorrow, and those with reduced *vata* energy.

FOOD CATEGORIES

IT HAS BEEN OBSERVED that the mind conforms to one of three categories – *sattvic* (pure), *rajasic* (stimulating) and *tamasic* (base and ignorant) – (see page 37). In Ayurveda, food is described as falling into the same categories.

Modern food science recognises that food is either acid- or alkali-producing. On the whole, most people eat acidic foods which cause deposits of free radicals (loose particles of oxygen which act on the body like rust on a car) and may cause conditions such as rheumatism and arthritis. An alkaline diet is more healthy. Ayurveda has a more sophisticated approach, defining food as *sattvic, rajasic* or *tamasic.*

Sattvic foods

Sattvic foods tend to be alkali-producing and are the highest-quality substances. They include fresh vegetables, fresh and dried fruit, salads, lentils, yoghurt, milk, fresh butter, wheat, rye, barley, hazelnuts, almonds, rice (especially brown) and honey. *Sattvic* foods help to maintain the body's health, increase strength, vigour and vitality, create physical balance (by maintaining the correct acid/alkali balance), and improve mental function and spirituality.

Rajasic foods

Rajasic foods are of medium quality. They are high in protein and generate high levels of physical energy. They include sugar, sweets, meat, cheese, fish, fried foods, eggs, potatoes and other root vegetables. *Rajasic* foods are deemed suitable for adults up to the age of about forty-five. Anyone over fifty should try to adapt to a *sattvic* diet as far as possible. Until the age of about fifty, the body has remarkable powers of recovery, but after this age the accumulation of toxins and *ama* (see page 42) increases and the system finds it increasingly difficult to cope with heavy and hard-to-digest food. All spare energy is needed to keep the body as well and fit as possible. (A specific branch of Ayurveda, called *Rasayana,* is devoted to rejuvenation. *Sattvic* foods are highly recommended for 'keeping us young'; *rajasic* and *tamasic* foods, on the other hand, have an ageing effect as many of them are processed.)

Tamasic foods

Tamasic foods are of low quality and include any which can be described as dried (except fruit), tinned, processed, spoiled (that is, cooked and kept), contaminated or junk food. All alcohol is *tamasic,* as are pharmaceutical drugs, tobacco, sweet, fizzy, manufactured drinks and snack food such as popcorn, crisps, salty nibbles, chocolate ice cream, and food containing preservatives and other chemicals. Illegal substances are *tamasic.* All of these damage health, cause physical imbalance and impair mental function. They can lead to personality disorders, such as hyperactivity in children, and should be avoided totally if possible.

Food and the *doshas*

All foods also have *vata, pitta* and *kapha* qualities and everybody's diet should take account of the prevailing *dosha.* Working out the right diet for someone can be quite complicated, so consult an Ayurvedic practitioner and get it right from the start.

Research into 'mood food'

Through its research into 'mood food' the Institute of Food Research in the UK identified two types of personality: the relaxed or satiated type (which corresponds to the *sattvic* personality) and the hard-working or aroused type (which corresponds to the *rajasic* personality). This report, *Peak Performance Living* by Dr Joel Robertson (1996), concluded that different personalities benefitted from personally tailored diets. Ayurveda has advocated this for thousands of years.

Meat, fish and eggs

Ayurveda recommends a vegetarian diet, so meat is not usually on the menu. However, if the practitioner recognises that the protein content of meat is appropriate in particular cases, the following properties are acknowledged:

✦ Beef is suitable for treating *vata*-related ailments, such as degenerative conditions, aching bones and tuberculosis. It helps to control an excessive appetite and encourages muscular growth.

✦ Lamb and fish (both high in nutrients) are heavy to digest, generate heat, increase growth and strength and reduce excess *vata.*

✦ Pork is heavy to digest, increases growth, strength and fatty tissue, and promotes sweating.

✦ Eggs increase lung capacity and sperm count and reduce the risk of heart disease (contrary to the view taken by most heart specialists) and the incidence of ulcers.

AGNI (METABOLISM)

THE SANSKRIT WORD *agni* means 'fire' and is used to describe the forces which break down the substances we consume. It embraces not only the enzymes and acids involved in the digestive process, but also the liver, gall bladder, salivary glands, pancreas and all the other organs and tissues which have a part to play in the creation and control of appetite and elimination.

Agni is present in every cell of the body. It maintains the immune system and destroys harmful bacteria and toxins. It protects the intestinal flora and the beneficial bacteria, which aid the breaking down of food into useful and waste products. (A disadvantage of antibiotics is that they destroy not only harmful bacteria, but also the body's own essential flora, a vital part of the process of *agni*.)

A question of balance

The proper digestion of food depends upon a well-balanced *agni* which in turn depends upon *dosha* balance, the right mental attitude to appetite and food intake, and the correct quantity of food. Long life, happiness and a positive approach to life also require a balanced *agni*. If its function is impaired, food remains undigested and unabsorbed, and accumulates as *ama* (see page 42). Toxins enter the blood supply and may cause illness and disease. (Orthodox medicine is showing an increasing interest in the harm which accumulated toxic materials can do to the body.)

It is believed that blocked *agni* can also be caused by suppressed emotions. Some of those who care for cancer patients believe that giving free rein to the emotions and having a positive attitude can, along with conventional treatments, lessen suffering and aid recovery. It is thought that unexpressed anger causes changes to the function of the gall bladder and food cannot be properly digested and a complex chain of chemical malfunctions follows.

Ayurveda recommends that neither the emotions, nor a specified number of bodily functions (see page 60) should be suppressed.

Transportation channels

Pathways, or channels, along which any substance within the body is transported are known as *srothas*. The human body is full of *srothas,* the gastro-intestinal tract being the largest. Their function is to move *doshas,* nutritional matter and waste products from one site in the body to another. This process should not be impeded. If the channels become blocked, efficient digestion is impossible and a disease process may set in. A number of factors may cause the channels to be blocked – there may be injury, the *doshas* may be out of balance, there may have been a shock to the system (e.g., an accident) or mental trauma (such as a bereavement). The patient may not be aware of the blockage of their *srotha* – in Western medicine, the symptoms which patients complain of are often the end product of this disorder: in other words, by the time pain or discomfort is experienced, the resultant disease process may have been established for some time. Ayurveda's aim is to ensure that the *srothas* do not become blocked in the first place, and that a disease process cannot take hold.

APPETITE

THE NATURE OF our appetite and the way we eat profoundly affects *agni*. A balanced appetite is called *samagni* – the *doshas* are in balance, and digestion, absorption and metabolism are all functioning efficiently. Disease cannot set in. However, malfunctions can occur in the system if the appetite is disordered. Ayurveda identifies three categories of disturbed appetite.

✦ **Erratic appetite** *(vishamagni)* causes the *vata dosha* to become unbalanced and can cause the following symptoms: distended belly; a feeling of fullness (even if little food has been consumed); abdominal discomfort or pain; constipation or diarrhoea; tiredness after eating; a general feeling of heaviness throughout the body; slow digestion; belching; nausea; gurgling sounds in the stomach.

✦ **Excessive appetite** *(thikshanangi)* causes the *pitta dosha* to become unbalanced and is manifest as the following: eating large quantities in a short space of time; feeling hungry shortly after eating; very rapid digestion; sweating while eating; a diminished sense of taste and smell.

✦ **Lack of appetite** *(mandagni)* causes the *kapha dosha* to become unbalanced and can cause the following: eating too slowly; an inability to digest food; abdominal heaviness; low-quality fire in the *agni*; a feeling of heaviness in the head; breathing difficulty; nausea and vomiting; coughing; general debility.

All of these eating disorders can cause serious imbalances in the system and can be difficult to put right. With its emphasis on right diet and eating habits, Ayurveda aims to restore *samagni* and sees this as its first weapon in the battle against disease (see the case studies on page 104). The therapies which are designed to unblock the *srothas* and restore correct *agni* might be likened to the cleaning system in a city. When the drains and sewers are blocked, there are bad smells. If the body's channels are blocked, unpleasant odours emanate from sweat, urine, faeces and in the breath. All of these provide important clues in diagnosing how and where something is wrong.

Keeping age at bay

Agni changes as we get older. The young have a gentle metabolic rate which gradually increases. It is stable between the ages of about forty and sixty, after which it starts to slow down and the body's tissues start to degenerate. Ayurveda recommends therapies to slow degeneration and deterioration. These treatments include therapies designed for rejuvenation and sexual potency called *rasayana* and *vajikarana* (see page 101).

RECOMMENDATIONS FOR HEALTHY EATING

AYURVEDA'S STRICTURES ON the subject of eating properly balanced meals, at the right time and in the right pace, inevitably bring it into conflict with the increasingly popular activity of eating out, and a growing reliance on the delivery of ready-made meals to the home or place of work.

While it is not totally impossible to indulge

in either of these and still maintain the right diet, it is extremely difficult. A typical restaurant meal, however carefully chosen, is most unlikely to have been designed to cater for the individual with his or her predominant *dosha* and particular dietary needs. Because eating out is regarded as a 'treat', most restaurants, bars and cafes serve meals which are richer, sweeter and, often, bigger than the consumer would make at home. The atmosphere in a crowded restaurant is not conducive to a measured pace of eating or proper concentration on the food being eaten, and digestion is impaired. People meet in restaurants to be sociable and enjoy company.

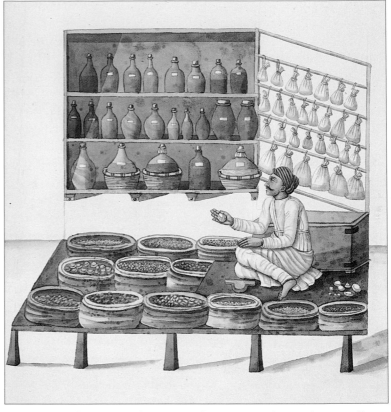

A nineteenth-century depiction of an Ayurvedic medicine seller.

One main meal a day

According to Ayurveda, the main meal should be eaten in the middle of the day, the luncher should concentrate on the food (and not read a newspaper, discuss business, etc.) and thirst should be quen-ched between meals, rather than through drinking liquids with food.

It is usual for appetite to diminish during illness. This is entirely natural and part of the body's defence against disease. Despite what some people believe, it is not necessary to eat 'to keep one's strength up'. Loss of appetite must, of course, be itself considered a symptom that something is wrong. If it continues for a long period you should seek advice.

TASTE STIMULATION

WE SAW THAT Ayurveda identifies six basic types of taste (see page 58). The tongue is covered with taste buds which detect different tastes in different places. Taste receptors respond to specific tastes. Ayurveda provides a 'missing link' by recommending a balanced diet which activates the whole metabolic system when the taste buds are stimulated by the six tastes. The proportion in which each taste should be provided varies from individual to individual, but Ayurveda cautions against a diet which is all salty, all sweet, etc. If some of the taste receptors are given nothing to do, they become blocked and ill health is likely to result. It is particularly important for children to be encouraged to eat a balanced diet – left to themselves, many would live on crisps and cola. The popularity of burger bars and similar fast-food oulets indicates that a diet high in fat and carbohydrate is worryingly popular among children and adults alike.

THE CAUSES OF OBESITY

AYURVEDA TAKES OBESITY very seriously and always tries to uncover the cause. Most problems stem from an over-dominant *kapha* energy. When there is serious overeating, the *vata* and *pitta doshas* 'go into reverse'. Low levels of *vata* acting on the thyroid gland cause the metabolism to become sluggish. A reduction of *pitta* leads to an accumulation of *kapha* in the fatty cells.

Water retention can also cause obesity and this too is believed to result from a *dosha* imbalance. A reduced influence of *vata* means that the driving force which expels water from the system is not activated, and *kapha* becomes over-dominant.

A further cause of overweight is lymph congestion. The *srothas* (see page 62) become blocked and toxins accumulate. There is not enough *vata* energy to drive lymph round the system and clear out the 'rubbish'.

Food addiction

Food addiction is becoming more common. Sweet and salty foods in particular seem to get people 'hooked' and they put on weight. *Sattvic* foods tend not to be addictive; *tamasic* foods almost always are (see page 61). Some *rajasic* foods can cause weight gain, including meat and meat products with a high fat content, cheese, butter, milk and fried food.

When people put on weight for no obvious reason, it sometimes emerges that they are eating more than they think or care to admit. If they continue to gain weight while eating a properly *dosha*-balanced diet and exercising, it is clear that all of the *doshas* have, for some reason, become very low and virtually inactive. Then a range of Ayurvedic treatment is needed to correct the influence of the *doshas*. An individual corrective programme will be devised for you by your Ayurvedic practitioner.

Comfort eating

Comfort eating is the term used to describe the consumption of types or amounts of food that have nothing to do with normal dietary requirements. This common problem, which can cause irreversible damage to the digestive and metabolic functions, can be attributed to a range of causes including: anger, stress, boredom, depression, bereavement, frustration, habit, failure in attempts to lose weight, unemployment, the breakdown of relationships and constantly being surrounded by food. To these psychological factors can be added impending illness or physical pain or discomfort. To make matters worse, the type of food eaten 'for comfort' is exactly the type which can lead to weight gain – chocolate is more likely to feature in the diet than cabbage.

FOOD TABLE

The food we eat directly affects our individual doshic state or prakruti. *Eating poor quality foods (see page 61), or foods which destabilise our dosha balance creates problems within the body. Pitta-types should avoid or eat smaller quantities of foods high in pitta, similarly vata and kapha types should be wary of foods which are high in their own dosha (see opposite).*

Your doshic state is also affected by the heating and cooling qualities of food, known as veera, or potency to perform action (see page 108), and many common diseases result from the wrong intake of heating and cooling food. Also eating the wrong kind of food can prolong illness. Vata types should eat moderate cooling and moderate heating food; pitta-types should choose cooling food, semi-cooked or uncooked food and veg-etables; and kapha-types should choose heating food, cooked food and vegetables. If you are a combination of doshas, e.g. kapha-pitta, you should mix heating and cooling foods in a suitable combination.

Your Ayurvedic practitioner will advise you on a diet which is suitable to your constitution.

Key

	Vata	Pitta	Kapha
High	▲	▲	▲
Low	▼	▼	▼
Level	◆	◆	◆

▩ Cooling food
■ Heating food

VEGETABLES

	Temp	Vata	Pitta	Kapha
Artichoke	■	▼	▼	▲
Asparagus	▩	▼	▼	▼
Aubergine	■	▲	▲	▼
Beans	■	▲	▼	▼
Beetroot	■	▼	▲	▲
Broccoli	▩	▲	▼	▼
Cabbage	▩	▲	▼	▼
Carrot		▼	▲	▼
Cauliflower	▩	▲	▼	▼
Courgette	▩	◆	▼	▼
Cucumber	▩	▼	▼	▲
Garlic	■	▼	▲	▼
Leek	■	▼	▲	▼
Lettuce	▩	▲	▼	▼
Mushroom	■	▲	▼	▼
Okra	▩	▼	▼	▲
Onion	■	▲	▲	▼
Parsley	▩	▲	▼	▼
Parsnip	▩	▼	▼	▲
Peas	▩	▲	▼	▼
Pepper	■	▲	▲	▼
Potato	▩	▲	▼	▲
Spinach	▩	▲	▲	▼
Swede	■	▼	▲	▲
Sweetcorn	■	▲	▲	▼
Turnip	■	▲	▲	▼
Watercress	■	▼	▼	▲

FRUITS

	Temp	Vata	Pitta	Kapha
Apple	▩	▲	◆	▼
Apple, cooked	■	▲	▲	▼
Apricot	■	◆	▲	◆
Avocado	▩	▼	▼	▲
Banana	▩	▲	▼	▼
Blackberry	■	▲	▲	▼
Cherry	■	▼	▲	▼
Dried fruits	■	▲	▲	▼
Grape	■	▼	▼	◆
Grapefruit	■	◆	▲	▲
Gooseberry	■	▲	▲	▼
Kiwi	■	▼	▲	◆
Lemon	■	◆	▲	▲
Lime	■	◆	▲	▲
Lychee	■	▲	▲	▼
Mango	■	◆	◆	▼
Melon	▩	▼	▲	▲
Orange	■	▼	▲	◆
Pawpaw	■	▲	▲	◆
Peach	■	▼	▲	▲
Pear	▩	◆	◆	▼
Pineapple	■	▼	▲	▲
Plum	■	▼	▲	▲
Pomegranate	▩	▲	▼	◆
Raspberry	■	▲	▲	▼
Rhubarb	▩	▲	▲	▼
Satsuma	■	▲	▲	▼
Strawberry	■	◆	▲	▼
Tomato, raw	■	▲	▲	◆
Tomato, cooked	■	▼	▲	▲

DAIRY PRODUCTS

	Temp	Vata	Pitta	Kapha
Butter	▩	▼	▲	▲
Cheese, hard	▩	▼	▲	▲
Cheese, soft	▩	▼	▲	▲
Cheese, blue	▩	▼	◆	▲
Condensed milk	■	◆	▲	◆
Cream	■	◆	▲	▲
Cow's milk	▩	▼	▼	▲
Egg white	▩	▼	▲	▲
Egg yolk	■	◆	▲	▲
Ghee	▩	◆	▼	◆
Goat's milk	▩	▼	▼	▲
Ice cream	▩	◆	▼	▲
Low-fat spread	▩	◆	▲	◆
Skimmed milk	▩	▲	▲	◆
Soya milk	■	◆	▼	▲
Margarine	▩	▼	▲	▼
Mayonnaise	■	▼	▲	◆
Yoghurt	▩	▼	▲	▲

MEAT

Beef	■	▼	▲	▲
Chicken	■	▲	◆	▼
Duck	■	▲	◆	◆
Goose	■	▲	◆	▼
Grouse	■	▲	▲	▼
Kidney	■	▲	▲	▼
Lamb	■	▲	◆	▼
Liver	■	▲	▲	▼
Partridge	■	▲	▲	▼
Pheasant	■	▲	▲	▼
Pork	■	▲	▲	▲
Rabbit	■	▲	▲	◆
Sausage	■	▼	▲	▲
Burger	■	▼	▲	▲
Tinned meat	■	▼	▲	◆
Turkey	■	▲	◆	◆
Venison	■	▲	◆	◆

SEA FOOD

Baits	■	▼	▲	▲
Breaded fish	■	▼	▲	▼
Cod	■	▼	◆	▼
Crab	■	▲	▲	▼
Fish roe	■	▲	▼	▼
Haddock	■	▼	◆	◆
Herring	■	▼	▲	▲
Lobster	■	▲	▲	▲
Mackerel	■	▼	▲	▲
Mussel	■	▼	▲	▲
Oily fish	■	▼	▲	▲
Oyster	■	▼	▲	▲
Plaice	■	▼	◆	◆
Prawn	■	▲	▲	▼
Salmon	■	▲	▲	◆
Sardine	■	▼	▲	▼
Shellfish	■	▲	▲	▼
Sprat	■	▼	▲	◆
Tuna	■	▼	▲	▼
White fish	■	◆	◆	◆

GRAINS

Barley	■	◆	▼	◆
Beans	■	▲	▼	▲
Brown bread	■	▼	▼	◆
Buckwheat	■	▲	▲	▼
Lentils	■	▲	◆	◆
Maize	■	▲	▼	◆
Oats	■	▼	▼	◆
Pasta	■	▼	▼	▲
Rice, basmati	■	▼	▼	◆
Rice, brown	■	▼	▲	▲
Rice, white	■	▼	▼	◆
Rice, yellow	■	▼	▼	◆
Rye	■	▲	▲	▼
Soya	■	▲	▲	▼
Wheat	■	▼	▼	▲
White bread	■	▼	▼	▲

NUTS & SEEDS

Almond	■	▼	▲	▲
Brazil nut	■	▼	▲	▲
Cashew nut	■	▼	▲	▲
Chestnut	■	▼	▲	▲
Coconut	■	▼	▲	▼
Hazelnut	■	▼	▲	▲
Peanut	■	▼	▲	▲
Pumpkin seed	■	▼	◆	▼
Sesame seed	■	▼	▼	▼
Sunflower seed	■	▼	◆	▲
Walnut	■	▼	▲	▲

CONFECTIONARY

Biscuits	■	▼	▲	▲
Cakes	■	▼	▲	▲
Chocolate	■	▼	▼	▲
Chutney	■	▲	▲	▼
Custard	■	▼	▲	▲
Golden syrup	■	▼	▼	▲
Jam	■	▼	▲	▲
Honey	■	◆	◆	▼
Marmite	■	▲	▲	▼
Puddings	■	▲	▲	▲
Sugar, white	■	▼	▼	▲
Sugar, brown	■	▼	▼	▲
Tomato sauce	■	▼	▲	▲

DRINKS

Apple juice	■	▲	▲	▼
Brandy	■	▲	▲	▼
Coffee	■	▲	▲	▼
Cola	■	▲	▲	▼
Hot chocolate	■	▼	▲	▲
Lemonade	■	▲	▲	▲
Malt drinks	■	▼	▲	▲
Mineral water	■	▼	▼	▼
Orange juice	■	▼	▲	◆
Tea	■	▲	▲	▼
Vodka	■	▲	▲	▼
Whisky	■	▲	▲	◆
Wine	■	▲	▲	▼

SPICES

Black pepper	■	▼	▲	▼
Cardamom	■	▲	▲	▼
Chilli	■	▼	▲	▲
Cinnamon	■	▲	▲	▼
Clove	■	▲	▼	▼
Coriander	■	▼	▼	▼
Cumin seed	■	▲	▲	▼
Fennel	■	▼	▲	▲
Ginger	■	▼	▲	▲
Mint	■	▲	▲	◆
Saffron	■	▲	▲	▼
Turmeric	■	▼	▼	▼

OILS

Coconut oil	■	▼	▲	▲
Olive oil	■	▼	◆	▼
Sesame seed oil	■	▼	▼	▼
Sunflower oil	■	▼	◆	▲
Corn oil	■	▼	▲	▲
Dripping,lard,suet	■	▼	▲	▲
Vegetable oil	■	▼	▼	◆
Walnut oil	■	▼	▼	▲

OTHER FOODS

Pickled food	■	▼	▲	▲
Salt	■	▼	▲	▲
Smoked food	■	▲	▲	◆
Stock cubes	■	▲	▲	▼
Vinegar	■	▼	▲	▲
Yeast	■	▲	▲	▼

WEIGHT CONTROL

AYURVEDA'S APPROACH TO weight control and its associated problems focuses just as much on patients who are underweight as those who are obese. Ayurveda also places great importance on treating weight problems as both symptoms and conditions.

While there have always been fat and thin people, there is no denying the fact that weight-related problems are on the increase. Greater prosperity in the West has meant that some people eat more (sometimes much more) than they need, and psychological problems are known to cause compulsive eating and comfort eating. Added to this is the fact that most readily available fast food is *tamasic* (see page 61) – the more we eat it, the worse it is for us.

An individually tailored diet

Conditions associated with weight loss, which have been identified and labelled relatively recently, include anorexia and bulimia. There are historical accounts of people 'starving themselves' – sometimes to death, but this tends to have been explained as an act of piety or asceticism (it often appears in accounts of the lives of saints). Some Eastern mystics were prone to demonstrating how long they could survive without food or drink. But Ayurveda concerns itself with today's problems as presented by its patients.

Ayurveda's approach to weight disorders is based on an understanding of the role of the *doshas*. A suitable diet can only be devised for an individual whose predominant *dosha*, genetic inheritance and *karma* are all identified. It is not enough, and is not even helpful, to offer generalised advice about calorie intake and exercise. The metabolic process works at maximum efficiency in the individual who is following the right diet. It is important to know which foods are easy and which difficult to digest. Appearances can be deceptive. Fatty foods slip down easily and are therefore mistakenly assumed to be easy to digest. Unfortunately, many convenience foods are high in fat, and there is a risk that developing a taste for such foods will lead to a loss of appetite for other, more easily digested foods.

Eating correctly

Ayurveda does not recommend dietary supplements or 'slimming aids'. Instead, it places emphasis on the individual the proper balanced diet for the individual. Although supplements may be recommended for people whose diet has become severely deficient, slimming foods lack bulk and can cause conditions such as irritable bowel syndrome, acute abdominal pain, haemorrhoids, gastric and peptic ulcers and diverticulitis. Appetite suppressants hinder digestion. Rather, Ayurveda recommends herbs and spices, as used in Indian cooking, because they stimulate the appetite and maintain the correct *dosha* balance.

Since ancient times, Ayurveda has recommended that we consume food of the six tastes (known as the *shad rasa*) each day to help our metabolism to function properly. Such a balanced diet contains all the vitamins and minerals needed to maintain health and strength, and is a much better regime than any attempt to take vitamins or minerals as supplements in isolation.

FASTING

FASTING CAN BE highly beneficial and some of its benefits are described below. However, it should only be undertaken with medical advice. Occasionally skipping a meal or even going one whole day without food may not do any lasting damage, but for some people it may not be advisable. It is always wise to consult a practitioner before embarking on such a programme.

People have fasted for as long as records have been kept. Historically, it appears that religious and spiritual convictions led people to deprive themselves of food, and it is still quite commonly practised – observant Hindus fast for one day each fortnight; Jews and Muslims have special times in the calendar when they fast.

Fasting can be an effective way of restoring balance in the system and of eliminating accumulated toxins. These surface very rapidly, causing headaches, nausea, spots, extreme fatigue and listlessness and an unpleasant taste in the mouth. The first day of a fast can be rather trying and unpleasant. However, such symptoms fade and the faster is left with a pleasant, light feeling. Fasting helps to unblock the *srothas* (see page 62) and improve memory.

Sensible practice

When fasting, it is essential to drink plenty of water during the day and when awake at night. The one-day-a-week fast helps obese people to lose weight, especially if it is accompanied by a move, on other days, to a *sattvic* diet (see page 60).

Some yoga and meditation organisations hold regular 'fasting weekends', which have the advantage of offering advice and supervision, as well as a chance to 'suffer together' with like-minded people. These occasions are highly recommended.

Obesity is not recommended. At best, it makes us uncomfortable; at worst, it can lead to ill health and shorten life. Heart and circulation problems and diabetes are universally acknowledged to be made worse by obesity. No healthy animal in the wild is overweight. An increase in *kapha* leads to lethargy and laziness. If an individual's dominant *dosha* has changed to *kapha*, it becomes increasingly difficult to lose weight as a vicious circle of overeating and weight gain is set up.

FOOD ALLERGIES

AN ALLERGY MAY be defined as the body's oversensitivity to substances which are not in themselves harmful. Some manifest themselves in obvious, visible ways (such as a rash); others are more subtle and cause toxins to accumulate in the system.

Ayurveda is frequently called on to treat patients with allergies to substances such as wheat, dairy products or shellfish, as well as to other everyday materials such as house dust or cat fur. Many people believe that the problem of allergies is on the increase because of environmental pollution and intensive farming, which often includes the use of chemical sprays.

Ayurveda's treatments include cleansing and detoxification (see page 90). Ayurveda cannot change the environment. But, by ensuring that the patient's system is as clean and free of toxins as possible, it can make a major contribution to health.

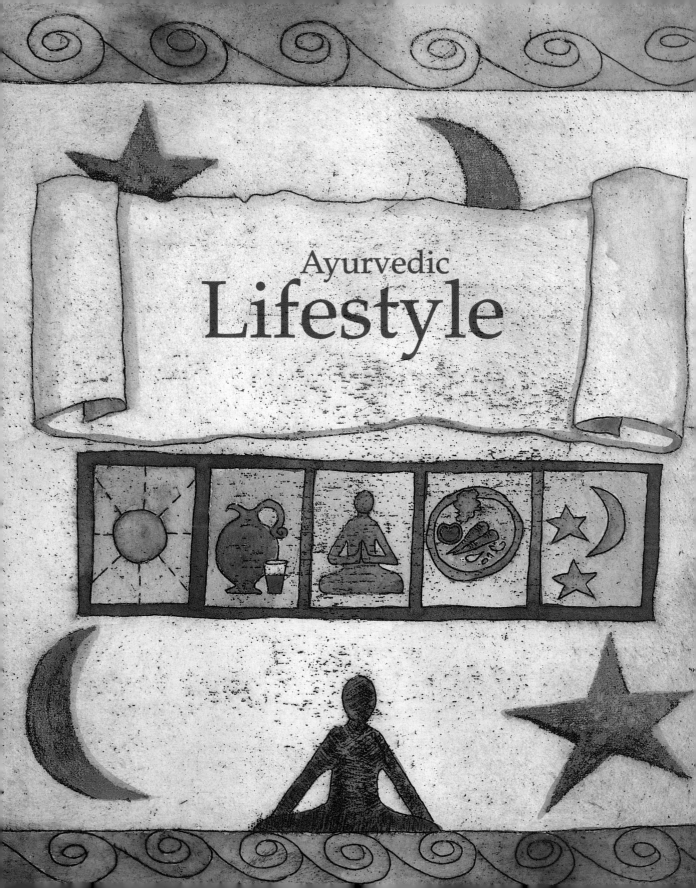

Ayurvedic
Lifestyle

Principally, Ayurveda is a complete system of medicine and people turn to it for help in treating disorders. But no system is effective if patients, before, during or after treatment, lead unhealthy lives which cause physical and psychological harm. The recommended Ayurvedic lifestyle is easy to follow and fits in with modern life and work patterns. It aims to maintain and, when necessary, restore harmony of body, mind and spirit without resorting to drugs which might have adverse side-effects. It encourages calmness and discourages constant, frenetic activity. Body and mind both benefit when people can adopt a meditative approach to life. Stress is a widespread and serious modern problem, not least because it suffers from being 'fashionable' in that there is a tendency now to blame everything on stress.

DINA CHARIYA

Ayurveda's recommended daily programme is called dina chariya. *Established thousands of years ago, it offers guidelines which, if followed alongside the recommended Ayurvedic diet (see pages 75–7), helps us to achieve whole new levels of well-being. It emphasises the importance of a daily routine which corresponds to the body's natural rhythms, and maintains calmness and harmony throughout the system.*

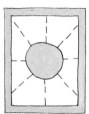

1 Try to wake and get up before sunrise. Most ancient belief systems stress the importance of rising early – in the West, there is even a proverb to make the point: 'Early to bed and early to rise makes a man healthy, wealthy and wise'. In the East, too, it is generally accepted that the body functions better on an early start to the day. In summer and winter, being up by six o'clock is recommended. Before you get up, spend a few minutes planning your day and thinking about what you want to accomplish during the day.

2 After getting up, wash your face with water and clean your eyes, nose and mouth. Scrape your tongue with a specially designed sīlver or stainless steel scraper (which can be bought from Eastern shops and is highly recommended). If the tongue is coated, food cannot be tasted properly. Clean your teeth with an Ayurvedic toothpaste and gargle with Ayurvedic oils or herbal preparations (which are on sale in shops which stock Ayurvedic products – see page 128).

3 Drink a full glass of water to activate the mechanisms for emptying the bladder and the bowels. Try to establish a routine whereby the bowels are evacuated at the same time every morning. Like all animals, we are creatures of habit, and our system works best when there is an established order of events. Constipation is a cause of many chronic complaints and a problem frequently encountered in the West. If people rush, they cannot give their bodies time to work properly, which is another reason for rising early and allowing sufficient time for everything.

4 In the East, the anus is always washed after bowel evacuation. A bath or shower is recommended following this function. It is important to wash the whole body every day to maintain a feeling of cleanliness and freshness. Ayurvedic practitioners believe that 'cleanliness is next to godliness', and this applies equally to body, clothes and the home. After bathing, Ayurvedic oils (appropriate for the individual constitution) should be applied; massaging the head with *neelyadi* oil can prevent headaches as well as baldness and greying and thinning hair.

5 Take some physical exercise before breakfast. Yoga is ideal as it is suitable for almost everyone (not just highly trained athletes), can be done anywhere and does not require special clothes or equipment (see page 79). Exercise improves the circulation and stabilises *dosha* balance. It enhances our capacity for work, both physical and mental, throughout the day. It can also powerfully counter depression.

6 Eat breakfast before eight o'clock. Wash your hands before and after eating. Clean your teeth and tongue after every meal. If possible, take some gentle exercise (for example, a 15-minute walk) to aid digestion.

7 Applying suitable Ayurvedic perfumes and wearing gems with special properties is recommended. A ring in particular, is traditionally believed to protect the wearer from the adverse influence of planets and demons. A more up-to-date view might be that we should take special care over how we dress, co-ordinating colours and styles so that our outward appearance reflects our inner harmony. The idea that particular colours suit particular people has its origins in the belief that we should dress in accordance with our individual *dosha* type, just as all other aspects of our lives should accord with our constitution.

8 Try to make lunch the main meal of the day. Eat the right amount (Ayurveda recommends that the ideal quantity of food for a single meal is that amount which can be scooped up with both hands), and at the right pace – neither too quickly nor too slowly. Be aware of the food you are eating: concentrate on it. If possible eat in silence, without talking or laughing – and certainly without arguing. All of these measures aid the metabolic process.

9 Do not drink with meals (except a sip of water to moisten the digestive tract). But drink water during the day. Avoid colas and other chemically manufactured drinks, and alcohol. Limit tea and coffee to not more than two a day. The correct intake of water varies from indiviual to individual.

10 Do not 'snack' between meals as snacking leads to an erratic appetite. Make sure that each meal is properly digested before embarking on the next one (on average, four to five hours, depending on individual constitution).

11 Do not smoke commercially produced tobacco. Ayurveda recommends, and supplies the materials for, therapeutic smoking (cigars containing therapeutic herbs), which can alleviate lung disease, coughs, hiccups, throat complaints, headaches, sinusitis, toothache, nasal problems, insomnia and general problems, such as loss of concentration and amnesia. Therapeutic smoking should be done after meals and after brushing the teeth. It stimulates the brain (whereas smoking commercial tobacco has the opposite effect).

12 Eat the evening meal early and allow time for it to be properly digested before going to bed. Whenever possible, go for a gentle walk (of around 30 minutes) before retiring.

13 It is time for bed. This is the appropriate time for sex. Ideally, lights should be out at ten o'clock. Do not sleep on your stomach, but try to sleep on your side with your knees slightly bent.

THE AYURVEDIC TIME CLOCK

10

2

Pitta
influence is most active between 10 o'clock in the morning and 2 o'clock in the afternoon and 10 o'clock at night and 2 o'clock in the morning. This is one reason why the main meal should be eaten in the middle of the day so that the digestive process is well under way by 2 o'clock. Gastrointestinal problems may become worse during this period and peptic ulcers can begin to bleed. This influence is not very active during the night because most people are asleep!

Kapha
influence is active in the period between 6 o'clock and 10 o'clock in the morning and the evening. Mucus collects in the mucous membranes and in the lungs. The movement of fat and the circulation of lymph are active and those patients who suffer from catarrh, sinusitis and asthma may experience difficulties at this time of the day. This effect lessens towards the end of the *kapha* period.

Vata
influence dominates the period between 2 o'clock and 6 o'clock in the morning and again is active between 2 o'clock and 6 o'clock in the evening. The end of this time in the evening is the best for physical activity and sport. Towards early morning, the brain is refreshed and this is the best time for thinking and planning. The best time for bowel evacuation is 6am.

6

The influence of the *doshas* varies depending on the time of day and night. Our bodies work to a time scale which ties in with the movement of the earth round the sun and, according to ancient teaching, with the movement of the planets. In classic Ayurvedic doctrine, it operates as above.

THE AYURVEDIC SEASONS

DOSHA INFLUENCE ALSO varies with the seasons; if our *dosha* balance is affected many *dosha*-related ailments can be caused. *Vata* influence increases in the autumn; *kapha* influence increases in winter and lasts until early spring, and *pitta* starts to dominate in late spring, when its heat can set *pitta*-type diseases in motion, including hay fever, rashes and summer diarrhoea.

The Ayurvedic year is divided into six seasons: *Shishira* (winter); *Vasantha* (spring); *Greeshma* (summer); *Varsha* (rainy season); *Sarath* (autumn) and *Hemantha* (the cold period before winter).

Ayurveda recommends that the body be prepared for a change of season through detoxification (see page 95) in order to promote good physical and mental health, and to alleviate chronic problems. No exact dates are specified, but rather a broad two to four week period at around the time the seasons are changing. It is difficult to set up a standard pattern of effects for the whole world because each geographical site may experience an entirely different type of weather at precisely the same moment. Also the pattern of weather during each season differs from country to country.

For followers of Ayurveda in the West, the recommendations on page 78 are offered.

SPRING

WITH THE APPROACH of spring, everyone should have some *panchakarma* (detoxification) treatment, then avoid strenuous physical activity and stressful situations for one to two weeks. This is a good time to take a holiday and relax, devoting time to the family and oneself. After a rest, it is advisable to take some physical exercise or play sports to a lesser degree than in winter.

◆ Continue with yoga and meditation every day.

◆ Exercise in moderation.

◆ Eat less heating and less heavy foods and continue with moderate to mild heating foods according to the changing weather conditions each day.

◆ Food with high levels of acidity should be reduced as they can cause inflammations or ulcers in the stomach.

◆ Sweets and a high protein diet are not required as the body does not require a lot of calories. A mixed diet with some carbohydrates, fat and protein is preferable. Anyone engaged in heavy physical work can increase carbohydrate, protein and sugar in their diet. If you are not burning enough calories, for example working in an office all day and travelling home by car, you do not require a rich diet. Stay slightly below daily calorific requirements (for instance, if you normally need 2,000 calories, reduce your intake to 1,800).

◆ Extra sleep should be avoided during the daytime.

◆ A warm bath of 10–15 minutes should be taken at least every other day.

◆ Wear clothes to suit each day. If the weather is warmer, wear light clothes or those which help to ventilate the skin.

SUMMER

In warm weather, and particularly when humidity is high, the whole body expands due to water retention. The cells retain more water naturally to conserve it for vital organic functions.

Pitta-related problems (for example, ulcers in the digestive system, gall bladder problems, infectious diseases and metabolic disorders) are common at this time.

◆ Prepare your body with *panchakarma* (detoxification) treatments. Blood circulation to the limbs increases and internal blood pressure drops and reduces the incidence of heart disease, strokes and other circulation-oriented problems.

◆ Sweat glands will be throwing out water to the skin surface to protect the skin from possible sunburn. Therefore, the whole external surface and all the layers of the skin are very active during this time.

◆ The requirement for physical exercise is reduced. Exercises and yoga should be kept to a minimum level and carried out in the morning (before sunrise) to maintain mobility and vitality.

◆ If you are working outside in extreme heat or sun, apply sesame seed oil or other specific, cooling oils prescribed by a physician to the whole body.

◆ Drink cold water and take food which does not aggravate *pitta*.

◆ Do not eat heating or very hot foods.

◆ Take more cooling food (such as salads) and plenty of cooling drinks.

◆ Eat a high-protein and carbohydrate diet which has a cooling effect. The amount of protein depends on the individual.

◆ A warm bath should last less than 10 minutes. If necessary, take a cold shower every day to remove sweat from the body.

◆ Walking under the moon is recommended during a hot summer.

◆ Alcohol should be reduced or limited to white wines. Spirits are more suitable in winter although they are *tamasic* foods.

◆ Reduced sexual activity is recommended at this time of year.

◆ Meditation should be carried out morning and evening, which has a calming effect and helps to avoid anxiety, anger and loss of temper caused by hot weather.

AUTUMN

Pitta-related problems are common at the beginning of the season, while *vata*-related problems start to build in late autumn.

◆ Again prepare the body through *panchakarma* detoxification.

◆ After treatment, take a break. Probably this is the ideal time for the main holiday of the year.

◆ Gradually reduce intake of cold foods and drinks as the weather gets cooler.

◆ Gradually increase your exercise and yoga programme or other physical and sporting activities.

◆ Eat a mixed diet comprising heating and cooling foods according to the weather each day, and also combinations of hot and spicy food with some salads and other uncooked food, and fresh fruit.

◆ Gradually increase the amount of acidic food while reducing the protein and carbohydrate content of the diet. Reduce the amount of sweets.

WINTER

IN COLD WEATHER, our bodies need to transmit additional heat (*pitta*) to our external parts. A drop in temperature causes the circulation of blood to the skin to decrease. There is also heat loss through the skin. The pressure on internal blood vessels and the heart increases due to reduced circulation to the external parts. The circulation to head and scalp decreases. Lack of humidity in the atmosphere can cause dry skin. Less physical energy is needed as outdoor activity is reduced. There is an increase in mental disorders - depression, memory loss, headaches - as well as in circulatory disorders, cold feet and hands, numbness and tingling, skin complaints, Raynaud's disease (a disorder caused by inadequate circulation to the hands and feet), aches, pains and rheumatism. The death rate from heart disease, strokes and hypothermia increases.

Eliminating toxins

In winter, waste products (toxins) accumulate under the skin and later travel through the circulation causing blockage of the channels (*srothas,* see page 62) and some organic disorders. Patients are given full-body massage with heated oils through the application of hot packs. During this treatment, all the accumulated toxins under the skin loosen up and increase the flow of blood, which disperses congested matter through the circulation. Meanwhile, lymphatic circulation is also unblocked and all the pores and sweat glands release toxins. After massage, patients are given herbal steam bath treatment which finally expels all accumulated toxins through the skin by sweating. Sweating and humid heat inside the heat chamber stimulate blood circulation and lymphatic circulation and leave the skin in a clean state. Most skin disorders are due to the continuous stagnation of toxins and bacteria in the pores. This type of cleansing complements internal detoxification (*panchakarma* therapy) and helps to keep the whole system healthy. A warm bath should be taken daily to maintain health; stay in the bath for 15-30 minutes.

It is advisable to take a tablespoon of honey in the morning as it improves immunity and energy and also breaks down excess fat. The following measures are recommended in winter (*vata* increases):

◆ Heavy, but digestible, food is suitable as digestive capacity increases.
◆ Eat heating foods (see page 66-7).
◆ Eat warm and cooked foods.
◆ Food with added salt and higher acidic content is suitable.
◆ Drink warm water and other warm drinks (such as tea and coffee).
◆ Vitality will be increased by taking milk, meat, honey, oil, rice and warm water.
◆ Oil should be applied externally.
◆ Saffron paste should be applied to the skin.
◆ Ayurvedic oil should be applied to the scalp.
◆ Sun bathing is beneficial.
◆ Warm clothing should be worn.
◆ Take daily exercise or play sports indoors, to improve circulation.
◆ Practise yoga and meditation daily.

**The seasons are not the same the world over –
dosha influence is affected by certain patterns of weather**

High temperature with hot wind	24–43°C (75–110°F)	P
High temperature with dry wind	24–43°C (75–110°F)	P, K
High temperature with humidity	27–35°C (80–95°F)	P, K
Moderate temperature, cloudy/ wet atmosphere	21–27°C (70–80°F)	P, K
High temperature, rain, high humidity and wind	27–30°C (80–90°F)	V, P, K
Mild temperature, heavy rainfall, no wind	21–27°C (70–80°F)	K
Cooling, comfortable weather, no humidity	18–24°C (65–75°F)	V, K
Very cool temperature with strong dry wind	4–18°C (40–65°F)	V
Very cloudy, wet, polluted air, smog	21–32°C (70–90°F)	K
Extremely cold with snow and ice	-7– -1°C (20–30°F)	V
Mixed rain and freezing weather	-4– 2°C (25–35°F)	K

Changes in *dosha* influence

Pitta-related problems are common at the beginning of the season, while *vata*-related problems start to build up in late autumn. *Kapha*-related problems (such as oedema, where watery fluid collects in the body cavities, general fluid retention, lymphatic congestion, respiratory diseases, asthma, catarrh and arthritis) increase during the rainy season and are therefore common in the periods before winter and summer.

The different stages of an individual's life are also dominated by different *dosha* influences. Childhood is seen as *kapha* time and lasts for about the first twenty years. During this period, children are susceptible to colds, coughs and asthma, which are all *kapha*-type conditions. From twenty until about fifty is the *pitta* stage, when the individual is most likely to be active and living life to the full as an independent being. Late middle and old age is the time of *vata*, when *vata*-type conditions, such as emaciation, breathlessness, arthritis, memory loss, wrinkles and dry skin, may be experienced.

It is believed that the body has great powers of recovery until about the age of fifty, after which things slow down. It is important to try to adopt a *sattvic* diet after the age of fifty (see page 60) and to reduce excessive physical activity.

EXERCISE

AS HAS BEEN suggested, every body needs the right amount of physical exercise for its individual constitutional type. The sedentary lifestyle, which is increasingly the norm, is injurious to health unless it is offset by regular exercise and exposure to fresh air. Lack of exercise can also contribute to stress and depression. And almost everyone can take some form of exercise. Ayurveda's approach is to recommend a programme tailored for each individual and, in common with its approach to other aspects of life and health, does not suggest that everyone needs the same type and amount of exercise.

Yoga

For Ayurveda, the best form of exercise is yoga which, happily, is becoming increasingly popular in the West. Although most people do yoga as a way of keeping fit, it was actually developed more than 2,000 years ago as an aid to spiritual enlightenment, by enabling *kundalini* energy to travel up through the *chakras* (see page 52). The word means 'union', originally implying union with the Almighty. At its heart lies the notion of gaining control – of the body, the mind and the emotions – by gentle but effective means. Yoga brings the body's systems into harmony; it increases suppleness and improves posture. Most forms of structured exercise practised in the West, such as aerobics and conditioning, have their base in yoga, which was the first logically worked-out system.

Ideally, we should get into the habit of practising yoga every morning and evening. If this is difficult, or if self-motivation and discipline are in short supply, yoga classes are recommended.

Yoga has two core aspects – *pranayama* (breathing) and *asanas* (postures). In recent years, research in British hospitals has focused on the benefits of yogic breathing as a way of alleviating conditions like asthma, eczema, high blood pressure and diabetes. The results have been positive. And there has been research into gentle yogic *asanas* as a means of dealing with serious back problems (one of the principal causes of absenteeism from work). It is essential that anyone with a problem attend a suitable yoga class, rather than trying to devise a home-made programme to deal with it. The Yoga Biomedic Trust was set up to investigate the medical and general health benefits of yoga.

Almost everyone can benefit from simple yoga exercises. Yoga does not require special clothes, though a tracksuit in winter and loose trousers and a T-shirt in summer are recommended. Tight, constricting clothing is not suitable. Remove glasses, contact lenses and jewellery before starting. Nor does yoga require a special location or equipment. It should be done on the floor – a bed or mat do not give the body the support it needs – and allowing a bit of space. A *sattvic* diet is highly recommended (see page 60).

Timing is important. Try to do yoga when you won't be disturbed and come under pressure to get on with something else. Ideally, it should be done on an empty stomach, before breakfast and before the last meal of the day are good times. On average, fifteen minutes on breathing and fifteen on postures is about right, but the Ayurvedic practitioner will give advice based on the individual's age, state of health and level of fitness.

Yoga exercises unlock tense muscles and restore flexibility to muscles and joints. Muscles are stiffer in the morning and looser in the evening. It is important to remember that yoga is not competitive. Everyone should practise those postures which keep them fit, supple and at peace.

PRANAYAMA (BREATHING EXERCISES)

IT IS RECOMMENDED that these be carried out while lying on the back, although they can be done while sitting or standing. It is important to keep the back and head in alignment (not arched or stooped). The exercises are:

✦ Complete breath
Breathe in deeply from the abdomen, which will expand, to the ribcage and up to the collar bone. Breathe out in reverse order and give the abdomen a gentle push to clear breath from the base of the lungs. Breathe in to a slow count of four, out to a slow count of four, and gradually increase to a count of eight.

✦ Complete breath with retention
Follow the instructions for complete breath above, but hold for a count of two between breathing in and breathing out. Gradually progress to holding for a count of four.

✦ Other breathing
For a count of four, breathe gently all the way to the diaphragm; this is very calming and may benefit angina sufferers. Inhale completely for a count of four. Exhale to a count of eight; this also has a calming and steadying effect. Follow the instructions for complete breath with retention. During retention, direct the breath to an area of pain or discomfort. After a few breaths, a warming sensation will be felt.

✦ Alternate nostril breathing
Place the right thumb on the right nostril and the fourth and fifth fingers of the same hand on the left nostril. Place the second and third fingers on a spot between the eyebrows. Close the left nostril and breathe in through the right nostril for a count of four. Close both nostrils and hold for a count of four, then open the left nostril and breathe out for a count of eight. Repeat, but the other way round, breathing in through the left nostril, holding, and breathing out through the right nostril. This technique is an important part of *pranayama* and is recommended for clearing the sinuses, and relaxing and refreshing the body.

✦ *Bhastika* breath
Breathe in and out completely three times. Inhale to one third capacity, exhale, inhale, exhale, and repeat for ten breaths using the lungs and ribcage like bellows. Finally inhale completely and exhale.

ASANAS (POSTURES)

YOGA IS DESIGNED to bring body and mind into harmony. Whatever is done with the right side of the body must be done with the left. For every posture, there is a counter-posture. Here are some simple asanas – do seek professional advice and guidance before trying them.

✦ The corpse
Lie on your back with your legs and arms spread and close your eyes. Turn your head from side to side, then bring it back to the centre. Remain still, then take ten deep breaths. Repeat until breathing becomes gentle and rhythmic.

✦ The easy pose
Sit upright with your legs crossed and pull your feet as close to your crotch as you can. Keep your spine straight. Roll your neck three times to each side. Rotate your head. If this posture is difficult at first, sit on a cushion.

✦ Leg stretches
Sit with your legs stretched out straight in front and together. Breathe in, raising your arms above your head, and stretch. Breathe out. Keeping your back straight, reach for your toes. Try to put your head on your knees. Repeat this exercise with one knee bent to the side and the foot against the thigh; then with the other leg bent. On both sides, and on the third repetition, breathe in, out and in again, three times. Sit with your feet and legs as wide apart as possible. Keeping your legs straight (backs of the knees on the floor, or as close as possible), breathe in and raise your arms above your head. Stretch and bend to the right while breathing out. Aim to touch your right foot with your left hand and lay your head on your right knee. Do this three times, then do the same to the other side. In the same sitting position, push your hands along the floor in front of your crotch as far as you can, and try to touch the floor with your head. You will feel a strong stretching sensation in the inner thigh.

✦ The locust
Lie on your stomach with your legs straight and aligned with your body. Keep your arms at your sides. Breathe in and, keeping it straight, raise your left leg as high as it will go. Breathe out and lower the leg. Maintaining a fluid movement and breathing freely, repeat with the right leg. Do this three times on each side. After the third repetition on each side, hold your breath for a count of four. Now try to raise both legs together while breathing in. Breathe out and lower. Relax the shoulders. Warning: if you experience pain or discomfort in the lower back when attempting this exercise, stop and seek advice.

✦ The shoulder stand
Lie on your back. Raise your legs together, supporting your back with your hands and with your elbows on the ground, until your shoulders are bearing your weight. Breathe in while raising the legs. Hold this posture for as long as you can. Breathe out when lowering the legs.

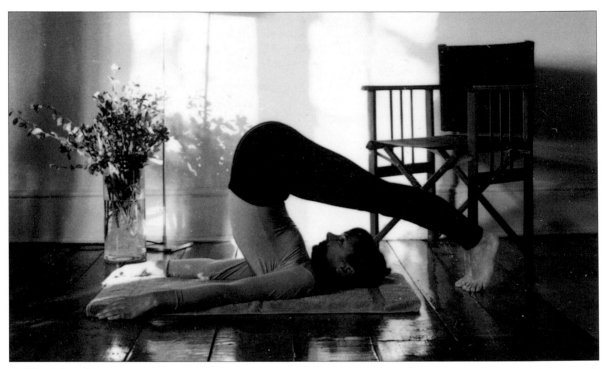

▲ *The 'plough' posture.* ▶

◆ The plough

Follow the instructions for the shoulder stand, but as you breathe in bring both legs over your head to touch the floor behind your head. Keep your legs straight and your arms by your sides. Breathe out slowly as you lower your legs. Repeat this exercise three times; on the third repeat, hold and take three deep breaths. Relax.

◆ The fish

Lie on your back with your legs straight and your arms by your sides. Arch your back until the top of your head touches the floor, but keep your buttocks in contact with the floor. Hold the position and breathe in and out deeply. Come out of the posture by sliding your head back to its original position until your back is flat on the floor. Relax.

◆ The tree

Use the wall or a table for balance when starting this exercise. Stand straight. Bend your right knee until your right heel touches your left buttock. Steady your balance, then raise your left arm straight up. Hold for as long as you can. Repeat on the other side. This exercise is particularly good for strengthening the stomach muscles.

◆ The final stretch

Sit with your legs together, straight out in front of you. Breathe in and raise your arms above your head. Stretch and breathe out.

Bend and reach forward, as far as you can, with your hands and chest. Sit in the easy pose (see page 81) for maximum relaxation. Breathe in for four and out for four, four times, then in for six and out for six, five times; finally, in for eight and out for eight, five times.

▼ *The 'shoulder stand' posture.*

Breathing exercises and yoga postures can help in alleviating specific complaints. If you suffer from high or low blood pressure, ulcers or asthma, ask your GP about yoga on prescription. A growing number of health centres now prescribe yoga-type exercises rather than drugs – which is a step in the right direction.

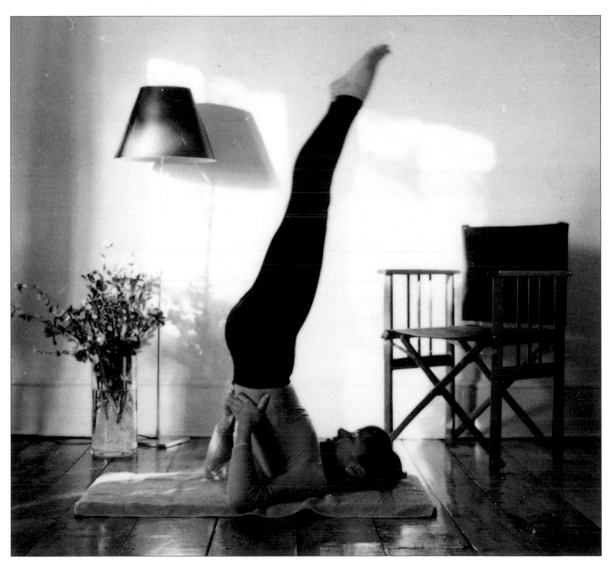

MEDITATION

BEFORE THE 1960s meditation was virtually unknown in the West. Then the Maharishi Mahesh Yogi introduced several well-known figures – most famously the Beatles – to the practice and it is now widely taught in health and leisure centres.

The best-known technique is probably transcendental meditation (TM), where one meditates on one's personal *mantra* (a Sanskrit word meaning 'instrument of thought' and a syllable, word or phrase which may be spoken aloud and as a chant) for twenty minutes twice a day. Another familiar type is autogenic training, which uses ancient meditative techniques to relieve stress-related conditions by helping to bring normally unconscious processes, such as breathing, under conscious control.

The benefits

In the West, meditation is principally taught as a way of reducing stress. Research has shown that it can slow your heart rate, diminish negative emotions and bring a general feeling of calmness to the system. It is always a good idea to try to get into the habit of meditating, however briefly, in situations where stress, distress or anger are present, or when an un-pleasant or frightening experience is faced. For a long time, people have been advised to keep cool and 'count up to ten' before speaking or acting in such situations.

Meditation also gives brain a rest for a few moments each day, revitalising it and allowing fresh thinking. Its benefits include heightened self-awareness; purification of the mind; emotional control; controlling anger; mind control; easing of tension; freeing the mind of clutter and obstructions, and improving memory and other functions of the brain.

It is understood that, in meditation, *kundalini* energy travels from one *chakra* to another in an upward direction (see page 52). This revitalises the organs and body functions corresponding to the *chakras.*

The gateway to enlightenment

It is also believed that, if practised for long enough, meditation allows us to read others' minds (telepathy), gain an awareness of our own previous lives, increase our psychic abilities and develop clear sight. In modern psychological parlance, meditation enables the brain to go into alpha mode, where creativity lies; normally, during waking hours, the brain is in beta, and in delta when we are asleep. Meditation is almost like a state between waking and sleeping, but with conscious awareness.

It works on the assumption that, at some level, we know all that we need to know. Within ourselves we have wisdom, power, love, insight and the ability to heal. We just have to find them. Insights and flashes of intuition can be achieved by a proper ability to look inwards. Meditation is increasingly being accepted as an effective way of purifying the mind, healing, and strengthening the immune

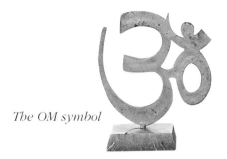

The OM symbol

system. At the Bristol Cancer Help Centre, where patients attend for counselling and gentle therapies, and where Ayurvedic treatment is offered, meditation is a key part of the approach.

Many people, who have never meditated, find it boring and difficult. Even a few minutes every day is beyond them. Their concentration lapses and they find themselves compiling shopping lists and wondering whether they turned off the gas and locked the car. But, with practice, these distractions become fewer and fewer, and as the meditative brain wave is reached, the whole exercise becomes very pleasurable and rewarding.

Often, it is easier to practise meditation in a group. And there are aids available, including musical and other tapes. For most of us, meditation does not come naturally and has to be learned. We have forgotten how to be still and sitting in silence can be a strangely uncomfortable and unnerving experience. It can also seem very boring.

For people who have mastered the technique, those moments of stillness and silence, when everything external is blocked out, bring a recognition of truth and an enhanced awareness of how things are, or how they could be.

HOW TO MEDITATE

Meditation is best learned from an experienced instructor. But there are a number of guidelines which can help you get started. Always try to meditate at the same time and in the same place each day. Breathe gently and with a regular rhythm from the abdomen. Start with five minutes of deep breathing, then breathe more gently. Keep warm. If possible, set aside a place where you will not be disturbed or distracted, and which is not used for any other purpose (eating, working, etc.).

Sit cross-legged on the floor with your hands outstretched, palms up. The eyes may be open or closed, but if they are open, focus on an object that you find relaxing and pleasing to look at or which has a special meaning for you. Try to focus your mind on a single thought, do not allow it to wander.

Choose your own special *mantra*. This can be a syllable, a word or a phrase, which you repeat, silently or out loud, as a chant. It doesn't have to mean anything, but should be simple. A common mantra is 'OM', which has a powerful vibrational sound when repeated over and over (see the symbol opposite).

Breathing meditation
(Anapanasathi-bahavana)
Try to focus your mind totally on your own breathing, concentration on inhaling and exhaling. Do this for 15 minutes in the morning and 15 minutes in the evening.

This method is highly recommended for patients with heart problems, high blood pressure and stress-related illnesses.

OTHER GUIDELINES FOR HEALTHY LIVING

✦ Rather than suppress a particular feeling or thought, get it out of your system by writing it down.

✦ Do not sleep lying on your stomach or your back. It is better for the body's energy centres to sleep on the side.

✦ Do not read in bed. This harms the eye-sight and fills the mind with active thoughts just at the time when it should be calming down.

✦ Do not try to disguise body odour with deodorants or other substances, but rather attend to the cause of the odour.

✦ Lie on your back on the floor, with your head resting on a couple of paperback books, for fifteen minutes a day. This brings the back, neck and head into alignment and is calming to both body and mind.

✦ Avoid addictive masturbation as it causes *vata* disturbance. Avoid sex during menstruation, as this also causes *vata* imbalance. During menstruation, women are advised to avoid strenuous exercise, including the more challenging yoga postures, such as the shoulder stand. Avoid oral and anal sex, which Ayurveda considers unnatural and unhygienic.

> Ayurveda believes that all human beings are meant to be cheerful, happy and positive in order to improve health and general well-being, both physical and mental, and to strengthen the immune system against illness and disease.

MEN AND WOMEN

IN CLASSIC AYURVEDIC teaching, the primary purpose of a sexual relationship between a man and a woman is to produce healthy children. Sexual pleasure and gratification are secondary. Because an individual's constitution and character are determined at the moment of conception, potential parents have a responsibility to ensure, as far as is possible, that they are in good health and that sperm and egg are of high quality. Preparation for having children should begin long before conception will take place, and Ayurveda has a number of recommendations for both men and women. (The Western approach tends to be not to intervene unless a couple experiences difficulty in conceiving.) These aim to maximise the father's and the mother's state of health, and to avoid having children with an already compromised immune system. Both are advised to embark on a thorough detoxification programme before conceiving.

Preparing for conception

The programme for both partners consists of the application of appropriate oils, sweat therapy, laxatives and therapeutic vomiting, cleansing techniques which will achieve proper balance of the *tridosha* in both sperm and egg. Following this purification, the man should include *ghee* (clarified butter) and milk in his diet, and the woman should include sesame oil in hers.

The woman should abstain from sex for three days following the end of her period. She should not have massage during this time, to avoid shaking the body when it should be stilled in preparation for possible conception. On the fourth day, she should bathe and wear white to represent purity. She should make sure she is calm and relaxed, and that she is eating properly and her digestive system is functioning efficiently.

The man should follow the same basic guidelines, and traditional Ayurveda recommends that he wear fresh flowers (e.g., a carnation in his buttonhole) to create an aura of freshness. The couple should then focus on the quality of their physical relationship, while concentrating their minds on their love for one another.

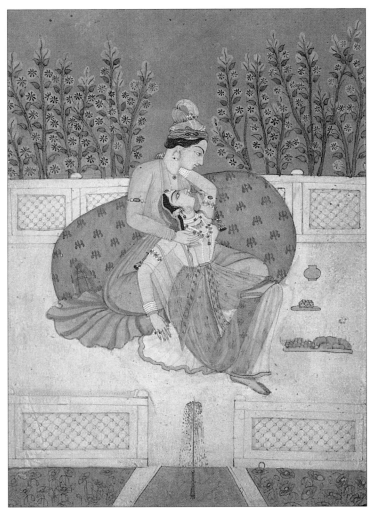

Indian lovers.

They should visualise the kind of child they hope to have, listen to uplifting music, look at beautiful paintings and scenery, free themselves from worry, and make themselves as attractive as possible.

Traditional teaching suggests that conception on odd-numbered days produces daughters and on even-numbered days, sons, but there is no guarantee that this theory works. Intercourse should take place with the woman lying on her back to increase the likelihood of conception. It is important that couples get to know each other well before they try to conceive. They should not feel disappointed by each other as this leads to their having negative feelings towards one another. Both should be free of any long-term illness. Neither should be too young or too old –

women should be fully mature and men fully potent. Men over fifty should not attempt to have children. There should not be a significant age difference between partners as there is an increased risk of birth defects and a weakened immune system in their offspring. Also, a significantly older partner is more likely to die while his or her children are still young.

Traditionally, couples have been matched by consulting their horoscopes.

Ayurveda teaches that character weaknesses in the mother or father can affect the unborn child adversely: a quarrelsome parent may give birth to a child who suffers from epilepsy; a man or woman with too high a sex drive may have to a promiscuous son or daughter; a worried parent may have a child who is timid, frightened and only has a short life.

Healthy parents make a healthy child

All of the above guidance is intended to enhance the health and happiness of the unborn child.

Once conception has occurred, the quality of the relationship between partners continues to affect their child, as does the quality of their thoughts. Eating an abnormal diet (for example, to lose weight), irregular bowel movements, taking strenuous exercise and being subjected to loud noise can all cause the woman to miscarry. What the pregnant woman consumes affects the foetus – in the West, pregnant women are strongly advised not to smoke and to drink alcohol very moderately. Research has linked illicit drug taking by pregnant women and a subsequent similar problem in their

children. Some studies appear to suggest that if expectant mothers eat peanuts excessively their children may be born with a nut allergy.

Lest it be thought that the whole burden of responsibility for ensuring healthy progeny falls on the woman, Ayurveda makes it clear that most of the same strictures apply to men.

Enjoying sex for pleasure within a marriage has been promoted in Vedic texts since the *Kama Sutra*. Good sex is considered by Ayurveda to improve the bond between husband and wife.

CHILDBIRTH

ACCORDING TO HINDU sacred texts, childbirth is the most important life event. Postnatal care is accorded the highest priority.

As mother and baby are regarded as a single unit, the father should not have sex or even sleep with the woman for the first three months after childbirth, reflecting the fact that, on average, menstruation does not recommence until that amount of time has elapsed (it may take longer). Those first three months are considered critical, and ideally the mother should be with her child at all times, feeding it, attending to its needs, and sleeping by its side. This is a counsel of perfection and women today are often unable or unwilling to fulfil this requirement. Now that infant deaths are less common, a more flexible view is taken of the three-month rule.

In the West, parents and their infant children are more likely to be separated than is the case in the East. Babies are usually put to sleep in their own rooms right away. Even in a hospital's maternity unit, mothers and babies are separated for long periods. Ayurveda takes the view that this separation deprives the child of its mother's warmth and touch, and induces stress, as indicated by much of the crying that babies do.

Breast feeding

Ayurveda advocates breast feeding and recommends that other methods should be avoided if possible. It is believed that breast-fed babies are emotionally and psychologically more stable than bottle-fed babies, and are more resistant to common infections. Traditionally in India, it has been taught that everything possible should be done to improve a mother's production of breast milk. Breast feeding is regarded as having religious significance and a woman's breasts are considered part of her 'wealth'. Herbal preparations have been developed to improve the quality and quantity of breast milk: *Asparagus recomusus*, *Withania somnifera*, *Glyvyrrhiza glabra*, *Trigonella foenum-graceum* and *Allium sativum*. Any of these may be given to women in the West who are having difficulty breast feeding. (There are also herbal remedies for infertility and to increase sperm production.)

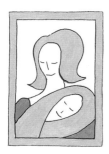

Child care

Ayurveda places the health and happiness of the child first. Conception, pregnancy and childbirth are viewed as sacred acts, to be entered into in a spirit of reverence, and not casually or carelessly. It is vital for couples to be compatible, otherwise they cannot create a happy home for their children. It is a couple's duty to have healthy children in a happy home – as little as possible should be left to chance.

Ayurveda in its strictest teachings does not look favourably on domestic arrangements which result in children being brought up by parents who are not their own. Ideally, if children cannot, for whatever reason, be raised by their natural parents, a close female relative would be first choice and certainly preferred to fostering or adoption by strangers.

WHEN THINGS GO WRONG

AYURVEDA MAINTAINS THAT sexual incompatibility is the principal reason why so many relationships go wrong. Traditionally, couples tried to avoid this pitfall by consulting an astrologer. However powerful the attraction between partners at first, incompatibility leads to boredom and restlessness. They will stray into having affairs, and what remains of their relationship is characterised by boredom and anxiety, rather than a balanced mixture of calmness and excitement. Infertility, in some cases, be attributed to incompatibility.

In Vedic astrological belief, there are twenty eight types of sexuality, some corresponding symbolically to different animals – e.g. the elephant, the deer and the cat. An elephant will not attempt to mate with a cat. Similarly, men and women who are not right for each other should not form a couple. But there is more to compatibility than sex.

Treatment

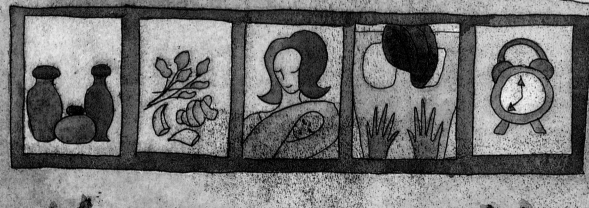
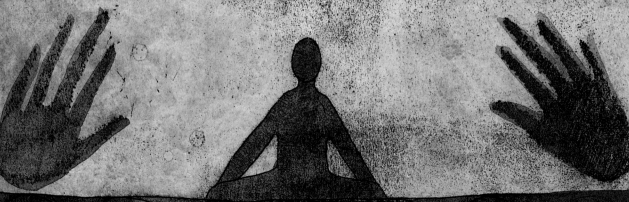

We have seen that the basis of Ayurveda is a holistic approach which seeks to take proper account of all aspects of an individual's health and way of life, and not to consider these in isolation and unconnected with one another. This is in contrast to the traditional approach among Western medical practitioners whose training inclines them to divide their areas of expertise into separate disciplines, and perhaps to see a condition rather than an individual patient coming towards them. Although some GPs do now try to adopt a more holistic approach, and are becoming more open-minded about the benefits of alternative and complementary therapies, most of their patients will expect a consultation to conclude with a prescription (very seldom without a warning of any possiblity of undesirable side-effects).

A VISIT TO AN AYURVEDIC CLINIC

THE AYURVEDIC DOCTOR treats the patient in a quite different way from a Western doctor. Before any specific treatment is offered, he or she will want to know as much as possible about the patient, including information about aspects of their lives which may seem to be wholly unconnected with the condition being described. As Ayurveda teaches that all treatment works best when the patient's system is clean, a detoxification programme is almost always the first measure. And, sometimes, it may stop there. Many modern conditions are caused by an accumulation of toxic waste in the system, and clearing that out often does the trick.

Treatments

Most Ayurvedic treatments are pleasant and patients can even find them enjoyable: 'no pain, no gain' is not in the Ayurvedic canon. All oral and external medications are herbal preparations. Some, of course, require determination (moving from a *tamasic* to a *sattvic* diet, for example), but the beneficial effects are often quick to appear, so encouraging the patient with an enhanced feeling of well-being and being well.

Generally speaking, the principal aspects of Ayurvedic treatment are diet, medication (to eliminate or neutralise toxins or vitiated *doshas*) and a daily regime, which should include meditation, yoga and *pancha-karma* therapy.

At first sight, an Ayurvedic clinic in the West might not look much different from a Western doctor's surgery. There is likely to be a waiting room, a receptionist, and even copies of the latest (or more likely, oldest) magazines. The Ayurvedic practitioner himself (most are currently male) will look pretty much like the average conventionally-trained doctor. But that is where the similarity ends.

Prevention

Where Western medicine seeks to cure illness once it has set in, Ayurveda is more concerned with prevention, with keeping illness and disease at bay, and with helping the patient to lasting, glowing, good health. To generalise, the most significant advice a patient is likely to be given is: stop whatever it is you are doing that is causing and aggravating your condition.

Illness strikes when body, mind and spirit are out of harmony. It is vital to consider both physical and psychological symptoms and seek out the connections between them. To look at either in isolation is to half-address the problem. 'Wellness', as defined by Ayurveda, is the body in balance and the body, mind and spirit in harmony.

The consultation

The first thing the Ayurvedic doctor will do, when the patient walks into the room, is establish the predominant *dosha (vata, pitta* or *kapha,* see page 25). While acknowledging that virtually nobody is going to display an undiluted cocktail of the characteristics of a single *dosha,* the doctor knows that the patient's dominant *dosha* affects everything else, not just the physical, but the mental and spiritual well-being too.

Having established the patient's *dosha* type – and a practised eye can do it almost at a glance – the doctor will feel the pulse (but not in quite the way the Western doctor or nurse does). In Ayurvedic practice, diagnosis of the *tridoshic* state is checked by three pulses at different points on the radial artery just above the patient's wrist. It takes years of experience to be able to understand the variations of the different pulses. Each corresponds to one of the *vata*, *pitta* and *kapha* energies and they are known respectively as 'the snake', 'the frog' and 'the swan'; the name reflects the principal characteristic of each pulse – sinuous, jumpy and smooth. The snake pulse has a high rate and is fast, strong and similar to the movement of a snake. The frog pulse has a normal rate and is warm, jumping, excited and irregular. The swan pulse has a slow rate and moves with a steady, thready, floating rhythm which may be difficult to sense. If any of the pulses seems abnormal, the doctor has his first clue about what type of condition he may have to treat.

The questionaire

Next, the doctor will ask the patient a lot of questions, initially about his or her parents and grandparents (the very people from whom we inherit our basic body type and constitution). What diseases and conditions have parents and grandparents experienced? If dead, at what age did they die? And what is or was their general state of health? The importance of this information is acknowledged by geneticists.

Ayurveda looks to the past for more than just genetic information. In India, where Ayurveda was founded, a belief in reincarnation and *karma* imbues every aspect of life and thought. In addition to a genetic inheritance, the patient also has his or her own *karma* - a cumulative legacy from previous lives (see page 16). The importance of *karma* is that it can override a genetic pattern – because someone's parents and grandparents died young of heart disease can be offset by a *karma* which predicates a long life. Ayurveda does *not* believe that we inherit a lifespan.

Questions about health

The doctor then finds out as much as possible about the individual's general state of health. Do you suffer from any chronic complaints such as eczema or asthma? Have you suffered any serious illness? Have you ever been involved in an accident or had a serious injury? Then there are questions about lifestyle to determine whether the patient's habits might be creating or exacerbating health problems. The doctor is seeking to make meaningful connections between the answers he gets and his reading of the pulses.

Questions about diet

Questions about diet and eating habits are of great importance. A basic tenet of Ayurveda is that the best way to lasting health is by eating the right kinds of food for the individual's *dosha* type. One of the greatest dangers to health is eating the wrong kinds of food. In general, Ayurveda recommends a vegetarian and high-quality diet, though acknowledges that non-vegetarian food may be appropriate in certain circumstances – reflecting the importance of not just offering the same dietary rules for everyone, but of also taking

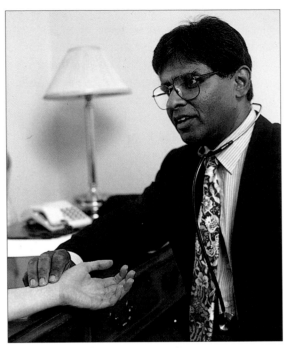

Ascertaining the patient's pulse type.

account of the individual's unique constitution. One of the principal aims is to prevent *ama* building up in the system (see page 42).

Questions about lifestyle

Some of the commonest problems Ayurvedic doctors treat in the West today are stress-related. Life in a post-industrial society is full of hazards – from an exclusively sedentary lifestyle to anxiety about job security – all of which impose a burden on individuals and families and lead to nervous collapse, marital breakdown and other distressing experiences.

Stress has a devastating effect on physical and mental health and has virtually replaced the scourge of infectious diseases with its own consequential conditions,

such as IBS, diverticulitis, ME, migraine, insomnia, Chron's disease, arthritis and skin complaints, all of which are difficult to treat. So the Ayurvedic doctor will want to know the answers to a lot of questions about the patient's particular circumstances and way of life.

Questions about social behaviour

There will also be questions about social behaviour and relationships – smoking, drinking and sex, for example. The first two may seem obvious and entirely acceptable; the third might be said to be none of the doctor's business if the patient has not presented with a sex-related condition (e.g., impotence) or a sexually transmitted disease. But Ayurveda has decided views about sexual behaviour and the consequences of breaking the rules. In the West, we are assailed by sexual imagery. Improper sexual activity, can lead directly to a range of conditions, not by any means all them sexually transmitted. Sexual activity should increase happiness, not end in misery.

Questions about symptoms

After all of these stages have been completed, the doctor will start to ask questions about the particular condition or complaint with which the patient has come – the astute practitioner will probably already have a very good idea what it is going to turn out to be. But the patient's input and his or her own appraisal are important in assisting diagnosis and deciding on effective treatment. After the symptoms have been described, the doctor will physically examine the patient – this examination differs quite radically from the type carried out by a Western doctor, and may include the eyes, nose, tongue, hair, nails, feet and skin. The tongue is particularly important in Ayurvedic diagnosis. It is believed that different parts of the tongue correspond to organs in the body. The doctor may also ask for a detailed description of the colour, quantity and frequency of your urine and your bowel movements.

A complementary therapy

A consultation and a diagnosis may take about thirty minutes to an hour. The next step is to work out an appropriate course of treatment. This is likely to be based on diet, medication and any necessary changes to lifestyle. It will be tailor-made for the individual patient.

Ayurvedic doctors prefer to work with, rather than in opposition to, the orthodox medical profession. A patient who has embarked on a course of medication will not be advised to come off it. It would be for the patient's GP to recommend stopping prescribed drugs.

Exercise is likely to be a significant feature of Ayurvedic treatment. Most people don't take enough, but it is important for the programme to suit the individual. Yoga is particularly recommended. Its purpose is not, as with aerobics, jogging, working out, etc., primarily getting and keeping fit, but rather balancing the body's energy centres, and bringing body, mind and spirit into harmony and symmetry.

Herbal medicines may be prescribed. These are natural and never artificially manufactured. They are the only medication in the Ayurvedic system.

All patients will be offered an internal and external detoxification and cleansing programme. Anyone suffering from a disease or complaint will have toxins in the system. Some of the techniques may at first appear strange to Western patients unfamiliar with them. But the programme is designed to suit the individual, and takes account of the health problem which has been identified. Before detoxification, oil massage and a steam bath help to eliminate impurities through the skin. The cleansing techniques described below must be carried out by a qualified practitioner. They are best undertaken early in the morning and on an empty stomach.

PRE-DETOXIFICATION
(PURVAKARMA)

Massage with oils (*snehana karma*)

This is the first cleansing treatment offered to most patients, and it is found to be enjoyable and relaxing. Depending on the amount of toxins that have built up, the

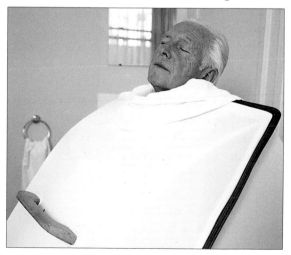

Patients find the sweat therapy very relaxing.

95

duration of each massage treatment may vary. In some ways, it resembles an aromatherapy massage, which more and more people in the West are becoming familiar with. The herbal oils are specifically chosen for each individual patient (using preparation techniques pioneered over 3,000 years ago), taking into account the prevailing *dosha*, overall body condition and the disorder to be treated. Oil massage is intended primarily as a form of medical treatment, its relaxing effects are secondary.

The most common oil is sesame, which strengthens the skin and protects it from fungal infections and the harmful effects of the sun's rays. Sometimes, a specially formulated *ghee* (clarified butter) is used, but plant oils are more common. Most Ayurvedic herbal oils have gone through rigorous manufacture based on original formulae. Apart from *ghee,* Ayurveda does not use animal fats.

The purpose of massage

Ayurvedic massage can be applied to the whole body and is designed to eliminate waste products, free up muscles and joints, improve the circulation of the blood and speed up metabolism. Gentle, circular motions are used, with the head and each part of the body being treated in turn. In treating women, it is important to include the breasts. No area is excluded, but due account is taken of any area of weakness, vulnerability or injury. Not everyone is accustomed to massage and the pressure used will vary accordingly. Frequency depends on the patient's condition and the severity of his or her disorder.

Following the massage, the oils should remain on the body for anything between 15 and 35 minutes, then the patient should have a warm herbal steambath for 20–40 minutes (see below). Immediately after this form of treatment, physical exercise, extreme cold, strong sunlight, shouting and giving expression to grief or anger should be avoided.

Sweat therapy (*swedana karma*)

This must follow oil massage. The Ayurvedic technique is more complex than a session in a sauna or steam cabinet, which many Western patients will be familiar with. Sweat is considered one of the body's waste products, a *mala* (see page 42), and its elimination can help the system to be rid of disease. Most people in the West do not sweat enough, through hard physical work or exercise, or otherwise. As a result, skin complaints are common. Sweating is also seen as unrefined – the manufacture and sale of deodorants and anti-perspirants is a multimillion-pound business. But many disease processes can set in when the body's natural processes of elimination are not working properly or are blocked. A lot of waste can be eliminated through the skin, and sweating keeps the pores open and the skin soft and wrinkle-free.

There are two types of sweat treatment: one initiated by heat (*agni*) and the other by external forces (such as exercise and clothing). Patients are always advised to increase sweat production, but they may also require a form which is activated by the physician. The procedure will depend on the patient's state of health and the nature of the disorder being treated. Heated gauze, towels, blankets or bandages may be applied to different parts of the body. Where there is swelling or pain, a warm medicinal paste may be applied. This treatment will not seem strange to anyone who has experienced spa therapies using seaweed, mud or oil.

A further method is to heat substances such as rice (usually specially cultivated for this purpose), sand, salt or mixed dried herbs, mix them with hot milk and apply in gauze bags to different parts of the body.

Finally, a concoction of medicinal leaves boiled with sugar may be poured into a bath and the patient is immersed in it.

Ayurveda advises against sweating only during eating. Food should not be so hot, spicy or heavy as to cause sweating.

Frequency of treatment

The oil massage causes toxins to rise to the surface of the skin; the sweat therapy helps to eliminate them through the sweat glands. Some patients may rest for 10 minutes and then take another steam bath.

Ideally, the oil massage and sweat therapies described should be carried out continuously for seven days. In most cases, this is not practical, and the interval between the two types of treatment and the frequency of treatment will be worked out by the practitioner in consultation with the individual patient.

General advice

During the external cleansing process, special care should be taken with diet and lifestyle as many metabolic changes will be taking place as a result of the treatment. Constipation should be avoided; drink boiled water mixed with coriander instead of tea, coffee, manufactured drinks and alcohol. Wear loose, light clothes to improve the circulation, and avoid strenuous exercise. Do not read material or watch television programmes which agitate the mind. A good night's sleep (6–8 hours) is essential. Abstain from sex and even from thinking about it. In short, avoid anything which imposes additional stress on the system. Have a warm bath every day and avoid cold baths, even in hot weather. The therapies leave the body and the mind in a delicate condition and their effectiveness will be enhanced by a calm and ordered life.

INTERNAL DETOXIFICATION
(PANCHAKARMA)

AFTER THE EXTERNAL cleansing treatments described above, the next step is internal cleansing, known as *panchakarma*. Some of the procedures will be unfamiliar to Western patients and may seem unpleasant and unappealing. However, unlike drugs, with their adverse side-effects, *panchakarma* treatments have only beneficial effects. Patients who are initially reluctant are surprised by how good they feel afterwards. The body is pleased to be cleared of rubbish. Ayurvedic doctors recommend a thorough cleansing four times a year, one for each season, as a general preventive measure and even if there is no disorder requiring treatment.

The five steps in detoxification are designed to eliminate negative *dosha* influence and accumulated *ama*. Appropriate for serious and chronic conditions, they must be carried out by a qualified practitioner and not all patients require all five.

✦ *Vamana karma* (emetic therapy) is induced vomiting. It is used to combat predominantly *kapha* disorders, such as indigestion, loss of appetite, chronic cough, asthma, catarrh, sinusitis and headaches. The patient's stomach is filled to capacity with liquids based on sugar, water and milk, and with a medicinal herb added to have the emetic effect. The patient's vomiting is supervised at every stage by the doctor and there should be a distinct feeling of relief. Patients should spend the rest of the day in as calm a state as possible, and avoid anger, grief, extreme cold and heat, strong winds, sleeping during the day, overeating and sex. Although this therapy sounds rather unpleasant, it is one of the most effective ways of normalising *kapha* energy. The Ayurvedic doctor may not recommend this treatment for Western patients because of its perceived association with bulimia.

✦ *Virechana* (purging) is used against *pitta*-related disorders. This therapy involves a herbal decoction which has purgative effects. It can be taken last thing at night or first thing in the morning. It can be done at home, but must be supervised by a qualified physician. After the patient's digestive capacity has been gauged. A number of laxatives will be prescribed and taken orally. After many eliminations, the colon is considered to have been thoroughly cleansed. This treatment is appropriate to combat skin complaints, asthma, urine retention, constipation, headaches and all toxic conditions. After treatment, patients should follow the regime indicated for emetic therapy above.

✦ *Anuvasana vasti* (oily enema therapy) and ✦ *Niruha vasti* (decoction enema therapy) are both administered through the rectum and differ only in the substances used, oil or herbal preparations. Both combat *vata*-related diseases and are considered the most important form of *panchakarma* treatment. They must be carried out in the strictly hygienic conditions of a clinic. *Vasti* is believed to confer happiness, long life, strength, power, intelligence and a positive outlook by eliminating toxic waste and *vata* diseases, which result from the retention of matter which should be excreted from the body. Conditions treated this way include gastric disorders, constipation, impotence, joint pains, headaches and convulsions. For women, some enemas are administered through the vagina and are recommended for patients suffering from infertility and gynaecological problems.

✦ *Nasya karma* (nasal therapy) is used to eliminate unbalanced *doshas* from the upper body. The patient inhales steam and medicinal vapour made from powdered medicines, dried herbs, medicated oils or the juices of medicinal plants. This therapy is used to treat catarrh, migraine, eye complaints, problems with the nervous system such as stuttering, and stiffness in the head and neck. It also clears congested sinuses, tones the face muscles and alleviates skin problems, loss of memory, paralysis and depression.

After cleansing therapy, an Ayurvedic practitioner will want to adjust a patient's lifestyle to bring recurring conditions, such as migraine or irritable bowel syndrome, under control. For serious disorders, a wide range of treatments may be recommended. When a disease has left the body, it can leave it weakened, and aphrodisiacs and other stimulating treatment may be offered to restore the body's strength. Yoga, meditation and daily relaxation techniques may also be prescribed.

Oil therapy – head (*shirodhara*)

For this therapy, the patient lies flat, face up, on a special wooden bed. An oil-filled pot with a small hole in the base is suspended above the patient's forehead, and a thin flow of warm, medicated oil is directed onto a spot between the eyebrows. The oil is then gently stroked down the hair for 30–40 minutes and permeates the skin. Sometimes the therapist will massage it in to the scalp for extra potency.

It can have dramatic healing effects. It is highly effective in the treatment of insomnia, migraine, epilepsy and amnesia.

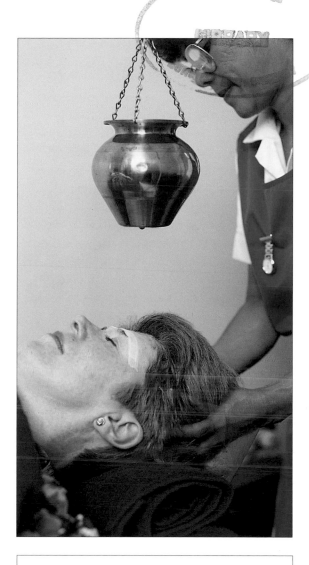

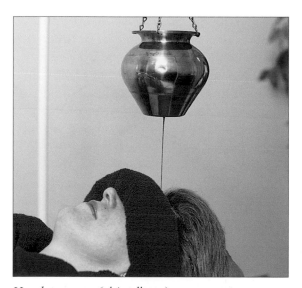

Head massage (shirodhara).

OILS RECOMMENDED FOR THE DIFFERENT *DOSHA* TYPES

◆ **Vata** – calming oils (sesame, olive, almond, amla, bala, wheat germ, castor)
◆ **Pitta** – cooling oils (coconut, sandalwood, pumpkin seed, almond, sunflower)
◆ **Kapha** – burning oils (sesame, safflower, mustard, corn).

HERBAL REMEDIES AND ORTHODOX MEDICATION

PATIENTS OFTEN ASK if Ayurvedic medicines are safe to take if they are also taking prescribed orthodox drugs. In most cases, it is perfectly safe, but a patient should always tell the Ayurvedic doctor about any medication being taken or that has been taken in the past. Several factors are borne in mind when Ayurvedic medicines are being prescribed: age, *tridosha* state, constitution, weight, body strength and appetite. And if the Ayurvedic doctor knows about orthodox drugs being taken by the patient, the dosage he prescribes can, if appropriate, be adjusted accordingly (modern Ayurvedic graduates are familiar with Western drugs as modern medical science is part of their training). By the same token, patients should always consult the GP who prescribed their course of drugs before they adjust or withdraw from the course.

THE IMMUNE SYSTEM

A RECENT ADDITION to the canon of Western medicine is psychoneuroimmunity (or PNI). It studies the effects of stress on the immune system and reflects a fact which has always been known to Ayurveda – that anything that affects the mind also affects the body, and that a compromised immune system is primarily the result of mental imbalance and negativism. Disease attacks when the *tridosha* are disturbed. If this point has already been reached, only vaccination has any chance of holding the disease process at bay, and drugs which are prescribed to fight the disease risk damaging the system, even when they appear to have been successful. This may explain why many people with undisturbed *tridosha* who live in infested environments do not contract diseases like malaria, hepatitis, yellow fever and typhoid.

To strengthen immunity, it is first necessary to improve the spirit. Someone who is depressed, lethargic and at a low emotional ebb is vulnerable to attack by pathogens. Similarly, unexpressed anger, unhappiness and other negative emotions leave the system open to invasion by illness and disease, as does exposure to a polluted atmosphere. Ayurveda does not believe in sleeping pills, tranquillisers or anti-depressants, which merely disguise the symptoms of a disorder and can leave the body even more debilitated and likely to succumb to infection. Instead, it recommends counselling, meditation, yoga, group therapy and herbal preparations.

When the *doshas* are seriously out of balance, two kinds of external disorder can take hold: *krimi roga*, which are worm infestations, and *kshudra jeevi roga*, which are parasitic, bacterial and fungal infections. *Krimi roga* disorders commonly afflict children and Ayurveda has special treatments to expel round worms, thread worms, etc.

Kshudra jeevi roga describes all other external complaints and includes infections such as chicken pox, mumps and measles. Unlike orthodox medicine, with its antibiotics, Ayurveda does not have treatments to kill these organisms but there are highly effective remedies available which restrict their growth and ultimately rid them from the body. These include treatments for malaria and hepatitis. It is accepted that they are part of life and we have to learn to live with them. They cannot be got rid of from the world. There are, however, treatments to alleviate the pain and discomfort associated with some of these conditions and strengthen the immune system by improving general health.

Ayurveda does not believe in attempting to create a totally sterile environment where such organisms could not survive.

If we grow up with them, we develop a natural resistance. It has to be recognised that man's battle with infectious diseases can result in organisms becoming more and more resistant to antibiotics (as has happened with the superbug MRSA – methycillin-resistant staphylococus aureous) and eventually the antibiotic will become ineffective. A better approach is to return to attempts to live in harmony with nature, and there is no better way to do this than by following the ancient principles and teachings of Ayurveda.

OTHER TREATMENTS

✦ **Rejuvenation therapy (*rasayana*).** It is important that every adult who has suffered from a long-term illness should be given full rejuvenation therepy. This involves some *panchakarma* and some specially formulated *rasayana* preparations. *Rasayana* improves the memory; and helps to maintain the mental faculties; helps to boost the immune system to protect against disease and infection. *Rasayana* also improves strength and vitality, the effects of which should be visible in the skin, hair, muscle tone, speech and performance.

✦ **Oral therapy (*shaanthi karma*)** has a long and well-proven tradition in India and Sri Lanka. When someone has been ill for a long time, and especially if the condition is of unknown cause and does not respond to treatment, an expert in oral therapy may be called in (every Indian village has one). The therapist strokes small branches from certain herbal trees to rid the patient's body of toxins and evil. Traditional Sanskrit or Pali phrases are chanted, and water is blessed and given to the patient to drink. (The therapy is also used for the dying. Buddhists believe that a disembodied spirit may attach itself to the living, causing harm, and may have to be helped to relinquish its attachment to loved ones and the world.)

✦ **Sound therapy (*manthra karma*)** is used to protect against ghosts and evil spirits. Special healing and blessing words and phrases are chanted all night. Good thoughts and vibrations can be directed at the intended beneficiary. (This therapy can also be used to inflict harm or even death. Harmful thoughts and vibrations are directed at the intended victim.)

In India and Sri Lanka, it is very common for politicians to use the services of such therapists. They may also wear a cylinder of blessed oil round the neck, or have blessed oil applied to the head for health and protection against adverse forces.

101

APHRODISIACS

(VAJIKARANA)

CLASSIC AYURVEDIC TEXTS teach that men and women are the best aphrodisiacs for each other. A woman should have beauty and good taste, she should smell good, and have a wonderful touch and a lovely voice – as well as a waist that can be spanned by two male hands and full-rounded hips. A man should also be attractive. Traditionally, it has been taught that it is more important for a woman to attract a man than vice versa, as survival of the species depends upon a man being sexually active. Women now feel equally entitled to sexual fulfilment, though it is not strictly necessary for producing children. While Ayurveda acknowledges changing attitudes, it can still fairly claim to be the first system of medicine that took proper account of the importance of sex.

Specific mechanisms which cause men and women to be attracted to each other include karma (see page 16) and availability (a very attractive man or woman is likely to have more choice).

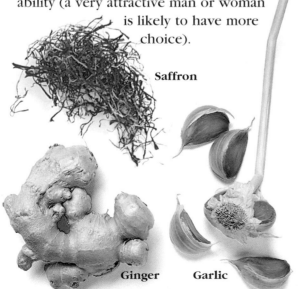

Saffron

Ginger   **Garlic**

All Ayurvedic aphrodisiacs are based on herbal preparations and are designed to 'awaken' the body. They are often prescribed to deal with infertility, impotence, premature ejaculation and frigidity and to increase sexual pleasure and virility.

Ayurveda is the only medical system to include aphrodisiacs in its pharmacopoeia. They may also be recommended when general energy levels are low.

ASTROLOGY

ASTROLOGY IS A branch of Vedic philosophy which works in synchronisation with Ayurvedic science. Planetary influence is accepted as a significant factor by Ayurveda. Humans differ from other living creatures only by virtue of the power of their brains; in every other respect, they are part of the planet earth and of the solar system. There is intimate synchronicity between what happens on earth and what happens in the heavens, and astrological signs, influences and portents cannot be ignored.

Although astrology does not form part of Ayurvedic treatment in the West, all practitioners are aware of its importance. The solar system must be kept in balance to work, and the forces which ensure this equilibrium are similar to those which keep people in balance. There is planetary influence in the creation and destruction of our physical bodies.

In most parts of India, midwives carefully record the exact time of each birth. In Sri Lanka it is a compulsory practice. Parents need this vital information for the astrologer who will suggest suitable letters to form

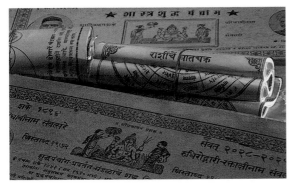

A personal astrological chart.

the name of their child (a child is not named until the eleventh day after birth), and will work out a chart which shows periods of planetary influence which may be expected during the child's lifetime. An experienced astrologer can predict much

of what an individual will experience in life. Time of birth is an important factor when it comes to matching marriage partners, whether the marriage is arranged or simply based on mutual attraction.

In India it is common practice to consult a Vedic astrologer when there is long-term or chronic illness, to determine whether or not the condition may be due to planetary influence. If it is deemed to be, the astrologer will make appropriate recommendations like wearing suitable gems and following certain health regimes.

As Ayurveda is founded on the concept of harmony between the inner and outer worlds, between earthly and heavenly influences, it views astrology as a legitimate science to be taken seriously.

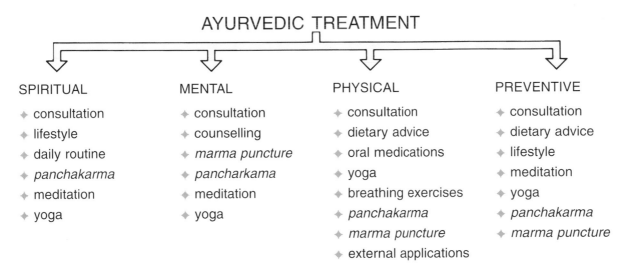

AYURVEDIC TREATMENT

SPIRITUAL
- consultation
- lifestyle
- daily routine
- *panchakarma*
- meditation
- yoga

MENTAL
- consultation
- counselling
- *marma puncture*
- *pancharkama*
- meditation
- yoga

PHYSICAL
- consultation
- dietary advice
- oral medications
- yoga
- breathing exercises
- *panchakarma*
- *marma puncture*
- external applications

PREVENTIVE
- consultation
- dietary advice
- lifestyle
- meditation
- yoga
- *panchakarma*
- *marma puncture*

CONTRA-INDICATIONS
Ayurveda recommends only natural herbal remedies and treatments and therefore there are few contra-indications. Many are based on common sense (e.g. pregnant women, diabetics, young children and the elderly should not take the purgative and emetic therapies of panchakarma). *It is important to remember that Ayurvedic treatments should be sought only from qualified practioner and that you should not withdraw from a course of prescribed drugs without first consulting your GP.*

CASE STUDIES

✦ Obesity.

Carol (45) went to her Ayurvedic doctor in great distress. She weighed 108 kg (17 stones). As with most overweight people, her obesity was due to addictive over-eating, rather than any hormone or metabolic imbalance. Orthodox medicine had not been able to offer a remedy. To help Carol get over her addiction, after a complete detoxification programme *marma puncture* was applied to *marma* points in her stomach, hand and leg. Her diet was modified to accord with her *dosha* type and a regime of fasting was recommended. As Carol's addiction was being addressed for the first time, she was able to stick to her proper diet and, within a year, she had lost more than 26 kg (4 stones).

✦ Anorexia.

Patsy (35) consulted her Ayurvedic doctor after suffering from anorexia for many years. She had received various kinds of hospital treatment and had nearly died on several occasions. Anorexia is sometimes called 'the slimmer's disease' and is believed to arise from a conflict between the body and the mind. Although sufferers may experience hunger, their resolve not to eat (in order not to put on weight) defeats the body's appetite mechanisms. Patsy's treatment had been based on attempts to get her to start eating again (including the use of drugs and 'reward and punishment' techniques), the Ayurvedic approach aimed to increase her lost powers of *agni* (appetite) and digestion by helping her to control her mind. Treatment consisted of counselling, preparations for strengthening the mind and oil massage of the head, diet, supplements, body massage and oral medication.

✦ Bulimia.

Lisa (23) was treated for bulimia. She was high *vata-pitta*. Bulimia is self-induced vomiting after eating. Causes range from attention-seeking to feelings of rejection, from self-loathing to excessive workload to stress in general. It mainly affects *vata*. The condition is characterised by binging, then vomiting and purging (vomiting can become automatic after a time). Lisa looked normal and was of average weight for her height. The first step was to prescribe herbal remedies to suppress the urge to vomit. Her treatment, which included anti-emetics and detoxification, returned her to health in six months. Ayurvedic treatment is based on a holistic understanding of the psychological causes of bulimia and of the physical and psychological problems which result from chaotic eating patterns. It has four components: restoring mental balance through counselling; restoring chemical balance with oral herbal remedies; restoring physical balance through exercise, and restoring all aspects of the patient through *panchakarma*.

✦ Allergy.

Carla (26) suffered from allergy, not just to different types of food, but also to cat and dog fur, petrol fumes, smoke and other everyday hazards. Her condition affected her mind as well as her body. Her food 'allergy' might have more accurately been called 'intolerance' as her body was reacting adversely to perfectly ordinary foods. Her treatment consisted of a cleansing and detoxification programme, and a diet of organic food. Now Carla's health is good provided she eats only organic food – before treatment, to test that the problem was not 'all in the mind', she was given some non-organic food but was told it was organic. She still had an adverse reaction. Once she regained her *dosha* balance she could eat non-organic food again.

✦ Eczema.

Anna (16) had suffered from severe eczema for at least five years, and none of the drugs or creams prescribed by her doctor seemed to help. She was often in severe discomfort, and sometimes had to have her hands bandaged at night to stop her scratching. With GCSEs coming up, Anna wanted to be as fit as possible and her mother took her to see an Ayurvedic doctor. She was a typical *vata* type, very thin, with thin hair and dry skin. She also had some *pitta* influence which manifested itself in cracked skin. At first she was not too enthusiastic about the recommended *panchakarma* (detoxification) therapy but agreed to give it a try. She had massage, sweat therapy and purging. She was advised to stick as far as possible to a *sattvic* diet (not easy for a 16-year-old, see page 60), and was given oral, herbal treatments. She was

asked to attend the clinic once a month for six months. After three months Anna showed a 75% improvement and after four months her eczema had completely disappeared. During the last two months of her treatment, there was no recurrence.

Extensive research into eczema has been carried out at the Government Ayurvedic Research Institute in Colombo, Sri Lanka, and the results have been excellent. There is almost always a dramatic improvement and, in many cases, a complete cure.

✦ Stroke

John (60), a solicitor, consulted an Ayurvedic doctor while suffering from the after-effects of a stroke. His right hand, the right side of his face and the right side of his body were almost totally paralysed. He had been told by his hospital that they could do no more for him and he was referred for physiotherapy at home. He feared that he would never walk again. Strokes are caused by over-dominant *vata,* and very powerful oils (*narayana*) and medications are prescribed to correct the obstructions in the nerve pathways which are causing the paralysis. John reluctantly agreed to *panchakarma* therapy (apart from induced vomiting) and, to his surprise, found that it had a dramatic effect. Because of the severity of his condition, John had *panchakarma* therapy regularly to open up his blocked channels, and followed a programme of suitable exercises. After eight months' treatment, his condition had improved out of all recognition.

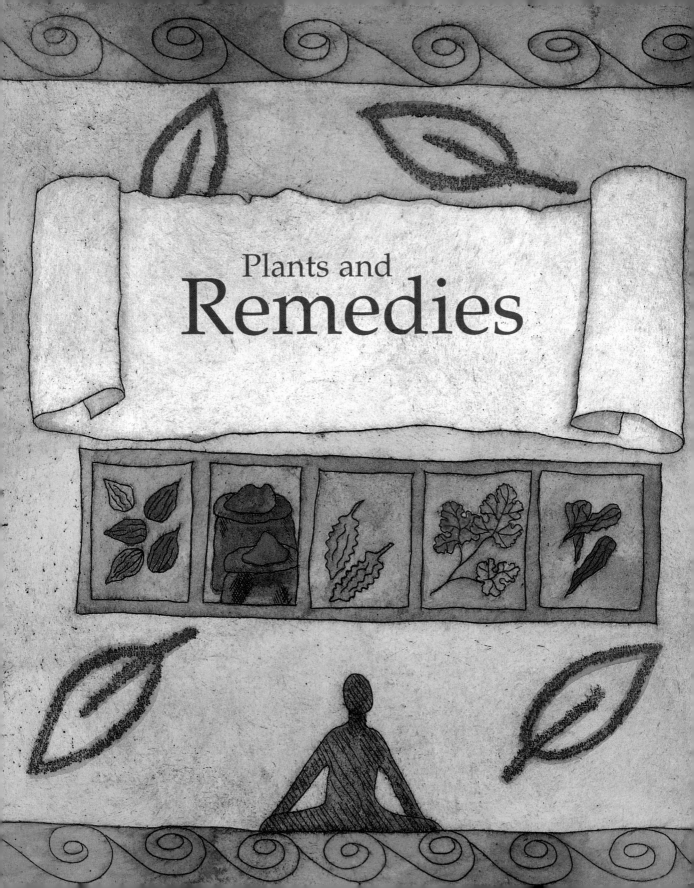

Plants and Remedies

Ayurveda may be said to be a treasure house of knowledge about medicinal plants. After correct diet, the use of the right medicines is the most important feature of the Ayurvedic system. All of the plants which are used for their medicinal properties have been thoroughly evaluated and classified for thousands of years. There are five key aspects attaching to medicinal plants: identification, cultivation, harvest, storage and usage. Identification is given the highest priority because of the importance of getting it right. Each plant is fully described in the Ayurvedic *Materia Medica* and is identified by the Ayurvedic classification system. Only then can the correct habitat, season and husbandry be worked out for the proper cultivation of plants.

In some cases the whole plant is used in an Ayurvedic treatment or remedy, in others only part; there are even prescriptions specifying that only plants which grow in certain direction are to be used; so collection must take place at the appropriate stage in a plant's development, and in the right season. Proper storage is important so that deterioration is avoided, with careful attention paid to how and for how long collected plants are stored. All plants are associated with the following properties and effects:

✦ *Tridosha* (the three *doshas)* – plants can be used to increase or decrease *dosha* influence as required.

✦ *Shad rasa* (the tastes) – every plant contains one or more of the six basic tastes (see page 58).

✦ *Gunas* (the properties) – these, in Ayurvedic teaching, are distinct characteristics which can be attributed to all matter, organic and inorganic, as well as to thoughts and ideas. The underlying belief is that everything in the universe is made up of a combination of opposing qualities. In ancient Chinese philosophy, these forces were known as *yin* and *yang,* coexisting as equal but opposite and unable to exist independently if life is to be sustained and continued.

There are twenty *gunas:* hot and cold, hard and soft, oily and dry, light and heavy, dull and sharp, subtle and gross, slimy and rough, unmoving and mobile, turbid and transparent, solid and liquid. The quality of any guna is impossible to know unless its 'opposite' is also present. The properties of each *guna* are related to the *doshas* (see page 25), and specific substances, which are characterised by specific *gunas*, can increase or decrease *dosha* influence throughout the body. The properties of each *guna* can affect the *doshas.*

(Confusingly, the three states of the mind – *sattvic, rajasic* and *tamasic* (see page 60) – are also known as *gunas.)*

✦ *Veerya* (potency) – every plant has the power to perform an action in two categories, hot and cold as does all food (see page 66–7).

✦ *Vipaka* (post-digestive effect) – after being consumed, the plant will be subject to digestive and absorption functions in the body and have particular effects on the system. After digestion the taste properties of the food may change.

✦ *Prabhava* (specific dynamic action) – this is the effect which the plant has when it reaches its final destination within the body.

A whole area of Ayurvedic knowledge deals with medicinal plants – *dravya.* This area comprises medication and dietetics.

Manufacture and prescription

All plants consist of the five elements. There are thousands of standard Ayurvedic preparations available today. Many formulas go through a long and difficult manufacture, and some preparations need to be fermented for more than a year!

Traditionally, physicians prescribed dried herbs for patients to mix and prepare at home. Today the commercial Ayurvedic manufacturing companies prepare liquid extracts and tinctures for every common Ayurvedic plant so that practitioners can stock them in their own clinics and mix various extracts and make compounds instantly for the patient. This type of practice is common and popular with patients and modern Ayurvedic graduates.

Apart from liquid preparations there are a variety of pills, powders and pastes available. Manufacturers follow strict guidelines. In the West, Ayurvedic practitioners can obtain preparations from India and Sri Lanka and some products are also available from specialist pharmacies (see page 128).

Possible effects

All plants can produce any of the following specific post-digestive effects in the body:

Blood purifying
Healing fractures and ulcers
Cleansing ulcers
Improving coagualtion to help
   stop bleeding
Breaking down kidney stones
Increasing appetites
Increasing bowel movements
Aiding digestions
Binding stools
Purgative and laxative
Expelling worms
Increasing or decreasing *vata, pitta*
   and *kapha*
Balancing tridosha
Preventing skin diseases
Reducing toxins
Strengthening the heart
Stopping fevers
Diuretic

The manfacture of Ayurvedic medicines is a huge industry in India and Sri Lanka. The Indian government and large private companies produce and distribute the products.

TYPICAL EXAMPLE OF THE PROPERTIES OF AN AYURVEDIC HERB

Sanskrit name,   Harithaki, a plant commonly used in Ayurvedic medicine

Botanical name   *Terminalia chebula*

English name   Chebulic myrobalan

Part used   Fruit

Special properties

Rasa	astringent, bitter, pungent
Guna	light, dry
Veerya	heat effect
Vipaka	sweet
Prabhava	effective in controlling all three vitiated *doshas*

Used to treat diseases caused by vitiated *doshas*:

fevers; infections; eczema; impaired vision; oedema

Form   decoction or powder

Effect   laxative or purgative

Harithaki is also used as a component of a wide variety of Ayurvedic medicines.

AYURVEDIC HERBS

MANY HERBS ARE used in Ayurvedic preparations, which are sold as essences, pills and potencised remedies as appropriate. Often they are herbs that are known and used medicinally in the West, although they are used differently in Ayurvedic medicine. Listed below are descriptions of some of the most commonly used herbs. The photographs were taken in a herbalist's Ayurvedic garden in Oxfordshire.

Plant name: *Cassia fistula*
Common name: Cassia pods
Habit: Tall, tropical shrub, to ht of 3m (10ft)
Used to treat: Diarrhoea, helps eczema – acts as painkiller.

Plant name: *Jasminum augustifolium*
Common name: Jasmine
Used to treat: Conjunctivitis, tetanus, ringworm and convulsions.
Habit: Native to Europe, Asia, Africa and US.

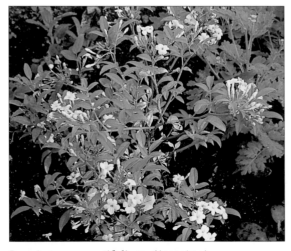

Jasminum augustifolium *(jasmine).*

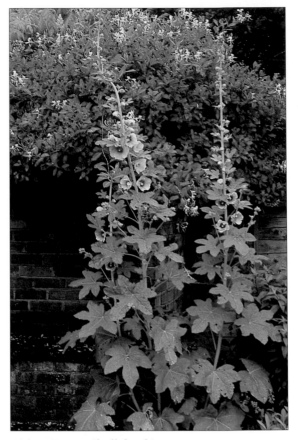

Althea Rosea *(hollyhock).*

Plant name: *Althea rosea*
Common name: Hollyhock
Habit: Popular garden plant
Used to treat: Irritable bowel syndrome; bronchitis; throat irritation; palpitations and cystitis – diuretic.

Plant name: *Citrus aurantium*
Common name: Bitter orange
Habit: Native to Spain, Sicily and the tropics
Used to treat: Bronchitis, asthma and indigestion – carminative, aromatic, anti-inflammatory and bactericidal.

Plant name: *Ficus racemosa*
Common name: Cluster fig
Habit: Hardy tree, to ht of 9m (30ft).
Used to treat: Unstable *doshas*, bleeding and colic–mild laxative, nutritive.

Plant name: *Helianthemum annuus*
Common name: Sunflower
Used to treat: Colds, flu and coughs
Habit: Easily grown from seed, to ht of 4m (12ft).

Plant name: *Zingiber officinale*
Common name: Common ginger
Habit: Easily grown from seed, to ht of 4m (12ft).
Used to treat: Arthritis, fevers, nausea, vomiting and asthma.

Plant name: *Coriandrum sativum*
Common name: Coriander
Habit: Native to Europe, Africa, Asia, naturally grown in N. America
Used to treat: Fever, diarrhoea and flu – calminative, anti-spasmodic, anti-inflammatory diuretic.

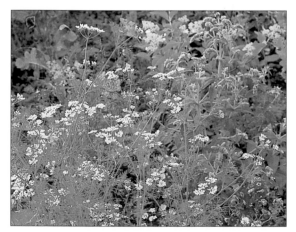

Coriandrum sativum *(coriander).*

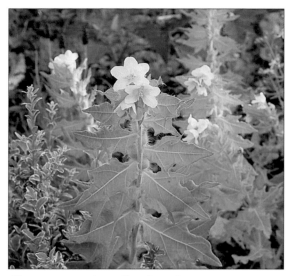

Hyoscyamus niger *(henbane).*

Plant name: *Hyoscyamus niger*
Common name: Henbane
Habit: Annual/biennial with yellow/brown or cream flowers, easily grown from seed, to ht of 80cm (32in).
Used to treat: Insomnia, anxiety, bowel spasms, colic, convulsions and incontinence – sedative and anti-spasmodic.

Plant name: *Kalanchoe lacinata*
Common name: Kalanchoe
Used to treat: Ulcers, abcesses and gall stones.

Plant name: *Datura stramonium*
Common name: Thorn apple – stramonium
Used to treat: Bronchial spasms, asthma, blocked sinuses and congestion.

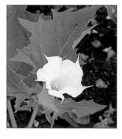

Datura stramonium *(thorn apple).*

111

CLINICAL RESEARCH

Ayurvedic plants have been tested in clinical studies with positive results.

Aloe vera (Kumari)

This is one of the most valuable Ayurvedic plants. It is used to treat a variety of ailments, most commonly bowel disorders such as constipation, diarrhoea and colitis; irritibility: gastritis; colic; skin problems like eczema, dry skin, itching, burns and cuts and feelings of irritability.

Aloe vera, a member of the cactus family, is a small bushy plant bearing green, fleshy, tapered leaves with juice that is very bitter and tart. Its medicinal use was widely known in many ancient civilisations including those of Egypt, Persia, Greece and India. Today it has been thoroughly researched by Western scientists. It is readily available in health food shops in the form of juice in bottles and gel in tubes.

The potency of *Aloe vera* is due to its rich variety of ingredients which include vitamins and nine of the ten most important amino acids, the essential building blocks of proteins. It also contains a wide range of minerals such as calcium, chromium, copper, magnesium, manganese, zinc and potassium; natural agents like saponins which have antiseptic properties; and anthraquinons which have antibiotic, anti-viral, anti-inflammatory and immune modulation effects.

The juice of this plant has miraculous healing powers. The active ingredient that plays a major role in this is the long chain sugar, B[1.4] linked acetylated polymannore. The B[1.4] linkage has proved to be particularly significant in that it plays an important role in the immune system's response to foreign agents as well as cell adhesion. The pathologist H.R. McDonald, MD , and his research team at the Dallas-Fort Worth Medical Centre discovered through their research in June 1993 that it is not only good for burns but also helps acne, allergic reactions, arthritis, busitis, colds, colic, candida, constipation, dermatitis, diabetes, water retention, ME, chronic fatigue syndrome, fungal infections, herpes (simplex and zoster), hypertension, inflammation, insomnia, indigestion, infections, menstrual cramps and irregularity, nausea, parasites, peptic and duodenal ulcers, psoriasis, reflex oesophagitis, sprains and teninitis.

Meanwhile Dr Jefferey Bland, PhD, formerly of the Linus Pauling Institute, studied the effect of *Aloe vera* on stools and bowel mobility for one week. His results suggested improved protein digestion and absorption and reduced bowel putrefaction. This change by itself could help prevent cancers in the colon. Further research by Dr Bland and his team discovered that *Aloe vera* juice has the natural facility to break down and loosen impacted material in the bowel which helps in detoxifying the colon. As this has no harmful or irritant effects on the bowel it relieves IBS (irritable bowel syndrome).

It was published in the *Medical World News* (December 1987) that Dr McDonald had carried out a pilot study on the effect of *Aloe vera* on AIDS (acquired immuno-deficiency syndrome) patients. He had been able to show that when 1000mg of *Aloe vera* extract was given daily to an

AIDS patient, the patient's symptoms were significantly reduced. Mega-doses of the *Aloe vera* extract were used in place of drugs and were found to be one of the most effective preparations when tested in conjunction with radio-therapy of patients with various malignant tumours. 'Andy', an AIDS patient, published a letter in January 1995 in which he stated that drinking the gel of this miraculous plant has helped to treat the 'morning sickness', a side-effect of the drugs he was taking.

Momordica charantia (bitter melon, bitter gourd or karella)

A research report published in the *Journal of Ethnopharmacology* states: 'The fruit juice of *Momordica charantia* was found to significantly improve the glucose tolerance of 73% of the patients investigated suffering from maturity onset diabetes.'

Well known to Ayurvedists, *Momordica charantia* is a commonly used fruit in India and Sri Lanka and research has shown that it is capable of stimulating insulin release that aids in: lowering blood sugars; tissue respiration; glycogen synthesis in the liver and muscle; and lowering fat levels in the body

Momordica charantia is also being used in America as a possible therapy for HIV infection. Dr Qingcai Zhang, MD, author of *AIDs and Chinese Medicine* (see Further Reading), has done some serious research work and reported positive results using the bitter melon treatment. It was reported that HIV positive patients were later found to be negative after treatment. Results showed that HIV cannot be grown on the cells of bitter melon-treatment-patients.

Research in America in 1990 observed that this plant protein is able to select and kill HIV-positive cells (*Compound Q Trichosanthin and its Clinical Applications*).

Allium sativum (garlic)

Purified and concentrated extracts of Garlic are being used as the controlling agent for PCP (pneumocystis carinii pneumonia) and for controlling sinus and chest infections which are common complications caused by AIDS. Garlic extracts are found to be very effective in viral and fungal infections; and also used for treating candidiasis of the gastro-intestinal tract and the many forms of unidentified diarrhoea.

Curcuma longa (turmeric)

This is often used in the preparation of Indian food often because it has the power to kill infectious organisms by destroying bacteria. It is still a traditional practice to preserve excess supplies of meat by applying a turmeric paste all over it which enables them to be cooked at a later date.

Turmeric is used in the household as an antiseptic and is often incorporated in commercially prepared phrameceuticals.

Research into Ayurvedic plants

A great amount of careful research into Ayurvedic medicine is constantly being carried out by the Government Institutions in India and Sri Lanka and by other companies throughout the world. The most important results are kept updated on database with the Ayurvedic Company of Great Britain (see page 128).

HOME REMEDIES

The kitchen is the most important room in the house – this is not only where food is prepared but it is also a potential domestic clinic. In the average kitchen many remedies can be found and prepared for minor ailments which work quite as well as expensive proprietary preparations. These ingredients can be bought from Asian grocers and supermarkets and, increasingly, from most large general stores.

Here are a few of the therapeutic uses for some of the most common herbs and spices.

Coriander

This pungent herb can be bought as leaves or as dried seeds. The seeds can be used in preparations to relieve sinus problems, headaches, colds and even cystitis.

◆ For *sinus problems* and related headaches: boil 4 tablespoons of coriander seeds in water and inhale the steam. Cover your head with a cloth or towel so that none of the steam escapes.

◆ For *colds and flu*: brown 4 tablespoons of seeds in a frying pan (making sure they do not roast or burn). Then boil the browned seeds in 4 cups of water with 4 slices of root ginger. Boil to reduce the liquid to 2 cups, strain the mixture and drink. A small amount of sugar may be added if desired.

◆ For *cystitis*: boil 4 tablespoons of seeds in 4 cups of water until the quantity is reduced to 2 cups. Drink this solution every day for a week. This will ease the burning sensation when passing urine, and will make it clear and alkaline.

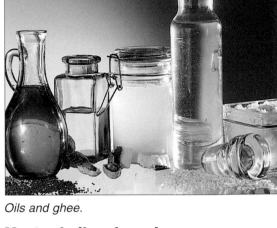

Oils and ghee.

Mustard oil and seeds

◆ For *headaches and fever*: heat 3 tablespoons of mustard oil in a saucepan. Soak a cloth in the solution and apply to the forehead. Dip the cloth into the oil at intervals to keep it moist.

◆ For *rheumatism:* mustard as a fomentation relieves aches and pains. Massage the body with upward movements.

◆ For *sore feet*: fill a basin with hot water and add 4 tablespoons of mustard seeds. Immerse the feet to relieve aches and pains.

◆ For *cold hands and feet*: massage them with a mixture of warm mustartd and sesame seed oils.

Curry leaves

◆ For *period pains*: combine 1 cup of curry leaves with 1½ tablespoons cumin seeds and 5 cups of water. Boil this mixture until it is reduced to 2 cups. Take this three times a day.

Garlic

Garlic, used extensively in Ayurveda and increasingly in the West, is effective in treating indigestion and relieving *chest pain* and toothache. Garlic in the diet reduces cholesterol levels. It also has anti-bacterial and anti-fungal properties.

◆ To treat *chest pain*: boil a few cloves of garlic in 2 cups of water until tender. Crush the cloves, mix with the cooking water, drink.

◆ For *toothache*: crush a clove of garlic and apply to the affected tooth. (An alternative is to fill the tooth cavity with a small piece of cotton wool dipped in cinnamon or clove oil.)

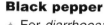

Ginger

Ginger is available fresh or as a dry powder. The fresh rhizome is more effective as a remedy; the powder, being more concentrated, should be used in small quantities.

◆ For *indigestion*: crush fresh root ginger to extract the juice. Mix with the juice of a lime and a lemon, and add a pinch of salt. Drink. Alternatively, chew a small piece of root ginger and swallow the juices which are released.

◆ For *coughs and sore throats*: crush a 5cm (2in) piece of root ginger to extract the juice. Add the juice to 1 tablespoon of honey and 3 tablespoons of lime juice. Sip four times a day.

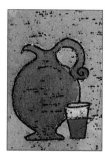

◆ For fungal infections in the mouth: rub the tongue with a piece of ginger.

◆ For a furry tongue: rub the tongue with a piece of ginger.

Black pepper

◆ For *diarrhoea:* combine 1 teaspoon of black pepper, 2 cloves of garlic, 1 tablespoon of cumin seeds, 5–10 curry leaves, a pinch of salt and 4 cups of water. Boil the mixture until it is reduced to 2 cups. Drink three times a day.

Butter or clarified butter (*ghee*)

◆ For *bee and wasp stings*; rub on the effected area.

◆ For *burning feet and hands*: massage with ghee or butter. Alternatively bath the body with fresh milk.

Karella(bitter melon or bitter gourd)

It is available from Indian greengrocers. The fruit is said to be tonic and calminative and good for the liver and spleen.

◆ For *mild non-insulin-dependent diabetes*: Boil and cut 1 karella into small pieces and eat, with the seeds. Repeat in the morning and the evening.

Lemon/lime juice

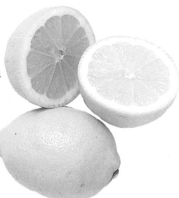

◆ For dizziness; add the juice of a lemon or lime to half a glass of soda water. Add some crushed ice if you wish. Sip in small doses.

CASE STUDIES

✦ Depression

Mike (45) was a hugely successful business-man and very rich, but had suffered for many years from depression. He found it impossible to sustain relationships and, since his divorce, had had a succession of short-term affairs, which ended with the woman leaving him. Mike thought he had it all, but his life lacked purpose and, rather than embark on another course of anti-depressants, he turned to Ayurveda. As Mike had taken drugs over a long period, his system was highly toxic. He started with detoxification, followed by oral medication, and physical and mental exercises including yoga and meditation. He also had counselling. Treatment took six months, and Mike was encouraged to adopt a more philosophical approach to life's ups and downs, and to break the 'habit' of being depressed.

✦ Osteoarthritis

Ellie (67) had suffered from severe osteoarthritis for more than ten years. She could not bend and was in constant pain. Her doctor had prescribed non-steroidal anti-inflammatory drugs, but her condition seemed to be worsening steadily. She decided to try Ayurveda. Her Ayurvedic doctor knew that Ellie's condition was caused by an accumulation of *ama* and *dosha* imbalance, and she needed complete detoxification and oral preparations. After two years, she is 75% free of pain and her flexibility shown an improvement of 50%.

✦ Impotency

Charlie (65) was very embarrassed to have to admit that he was impotent, but declared that he was not ready to give up sex just yet. Some *panchakarma* treatments were pre-scribed to clear obstructions and improve circulation, along with Ayurvedic aphrodisiacs taken orally. After four months, although not completely cured, Charlie was again able to sustain erections.

✦ Gastric ulcers

Nigel (49) was a dentist who had suffered from gastric ulcers for several years and was taking prescribed medication. He continued with this course while also having Ayurvedic treatment for his common, and predominantly *pitta* condition. He was given dietary advice suitable for his constitution and herbal prepa-rations to make his system more alkaline and to reduce stress. After six months a barium meal test confirmed that he had no ulcers.

✦ Irritable bowel syndrome (I.B.S.)

Catherine (34) had suffered from IBS for five years. Characteristically, she experienced abdominal pain, diarrhoea, constipation, flatu-lence and bloating, caused by *vata* distur-bance in the intestines. Catherine's Ayurvedic doctor prescribed pre-detoxification and some elements of *panchakarma,* particularly purg-ing. She embarked on an eight-month pro-gramme of treatment, which also included oral preparations, after which her bowel function had returned to normal.

CASE STUDIES

✦ M.E.

Eric (38), a teacher, had suffered from ME for several years by the time he saw an Ayurvedic doctor. He had been off work for six months. Complete detoxification was needed, together with oral preparations to strengthen his immune system. He also had *marma puncture* and followed an individually tailored diet which included some fasting. The aim of this treatment is to balance the *doshas* and, in Eric's case, was used to improve his appetite. After three months he was able to return to work. He still gets tired but follows as closely as he can the recommended Ayurvedic lifestyle (see page 69), which he finds particularly beneficial.

✦ Non-insulin dependent diabetes

Jane (18), a student, came to see me three years after she had first been diagnosed as diabetic. Because sugar levels in diabetic patients are difficult to control dietary advice is very important. Ayurveda also recommends oral preparations made from plants which act upon the levels of glucose in the blood.

Jane's *dosha* type is high *kapha*. I treated her with Ayurvedic herbal tablets, a dietary programme, exercise advice and *marma puncture*. After two months her blood sugar levels returned to normal and within six months her GP agreed that she could withdraw from her prescribed medicine. She is still stable and has not needed more treatment. She still continues to follow the dietary and exercise advice.

✦ Viral flu

Karen (35) is my neighbour and a dance teacher. She was one of the 10 million people in the UK who contracted viral flu in January 1997. She had been laid low for four weeks with nausea and a dry cough. Lethargy prevented her from going out. After a consultation, I prescribed a mixture of Ayurvedic herbs – *Solanum santhocarpum* (wild egg plant), *Adatoda vassica* (vasaka), root ginger and *Piper longum* (long pepper) – which was to be boiled in water and this decoction taken every 2 hours. I also gave her *marma puncture* treatment.

After about ten hours Karen began to feel better and within two day she was completely recovered.

✦ Anorexia

Sarah (26) was a nurse but had to give up her job when her anorexia, which had been developing over a six year period, worsened. Her Ayurvedic treatment focused initially on the recovery of her *agni* (digestive fire and metabolism) and a body building programme. She was treated with Ayurvedic preparations, *marma puncture* and was advised to practise yoga and meditation. Within six months of this treatment she regained her vitality and more than two stones in weight and she was eating properly again.

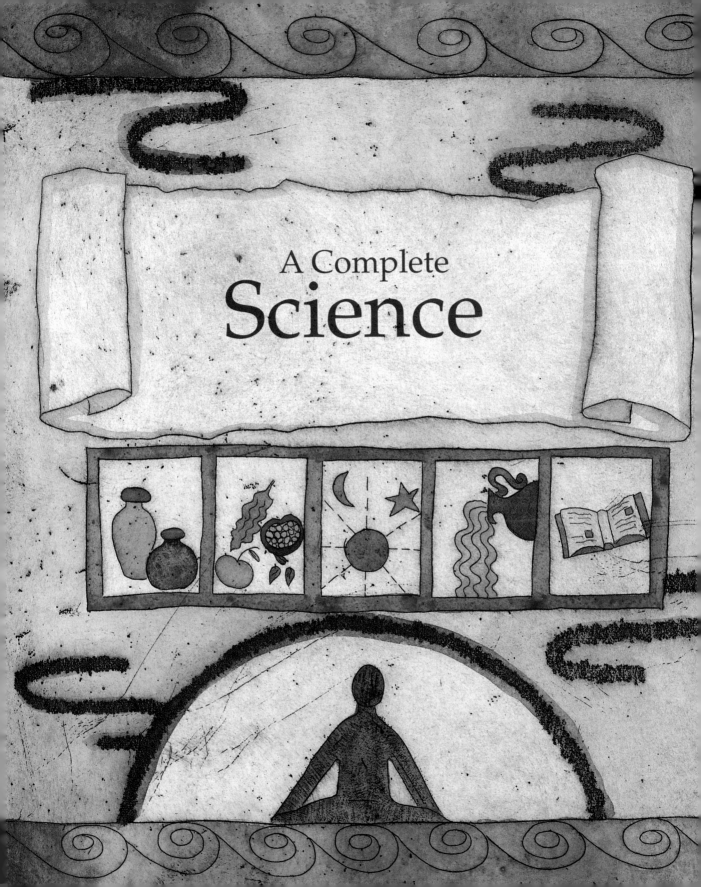

A Complete
Science

One of the most intriguing and appealing features of Ayurveda is that such a wide-ranging and all-embracing system of medicine can be like a precision instrument. While it is intuitive and creative, it has the logic and exactness of a geometric formula or an algebraic equation. If anything, however small and insignificant it may seem, goes wrong, the whole system cannot function properly. Ayurveda is based on this simple truth. A tiny imbalance can, over time, cause serious ill health. For example, a spoonful of sugar in a cup of tea three times a day may not seem life-threatening, but if the system is allergic to sugar, and inclined to obesity, the long-term effects can be extremely harmful. Similarly, bad posture may go unnoticed for many years, but ultimately result in chronic back pain and may even adversely affect other parts of the body, such as the heart, lungs and liver.

Because Ayurveda understands at a deep level and in great detail how and why things go wrong in the human system, physical and mental, it has been able to develop ways of putting them right. Equally important is Ayurveda's emphasis on prevention.

Treating the whole person

Although Ayurveda itself is still unfamiliar to most people in the West, and some of the terminology appears difficult to understand, those who discover it find it answers many (if not all) of their questions about treating troublesome conditions in ways which address not just a localised problem, but the whole person. Innate intelligence and knowledge of our own bodies can serve us well, but from time to time we all appreciate having a set of rules or guidelines to which we can refer if necessary. However clear we are about how we should live in order to maximise physical and spiritual well-being, modern life confronts us with innumerable obstacles and challenges which distract us and lead to our straying from the right path. This is why Ayurveda is gaining in popularity in parts of the world where it has not been a traditional part of the culture.

One of the things which distinguishes Ayurveda from orthodox Western medical practice is its focus on the person rather than the condition. Although several patients may display similar symptoms and attach the same label to their complaint or illness, each must be treated as a unique individual. The Ayurvedic doctor wants as much information as possible about every aspect of a patient's life in order to make a proper diagnosis, prescribe the appropriate treatment, and offer general advice about lifestyle which will help the patient to get well and stay well. A further benefit of this approach is that the patient too learns a lot about his or her individual constitution and what the indications are for enabling him or her to live a long and healthy life. There is no point in following advice which is right for someone else.

Despite the fact that many patients turn to Ayurveda when orthodox medicine has not given them what they need, Ayurveda does not see itself as working in opposition to, or in competition with, Western medicine. By adopting what is usually referred to in English as 'the holistic approach', it seeks to offer patients treatment and advice on a comprehensive basis, not just dispensing medication, but also offering cleansing and dietary advice, and recommendations for physical and mental exercise, tailor-made for the individual.

The vital role of Western medicine

Western medicine is impressive, with its array of high-tech equipment and its powerful drugs. But it can also be intimidating and sometimes the cure is worse than the disease. For treating medical emergencies, with or without surgical intervention, it is unrivalled. Any of us may be unlucky enough to be injured in an accident, and we look to the public or private health services to put us back together. But many people find themselves calling on the medical system to put right disorders that could have been prevented.

Some readers may have found the guidelines for healthy living described in this book somewhat daunting. But many people admit that, while they may not at this moment have a complaint which they can take to a doctor, they know instinctively that they do not feel as well as they could, and, if they stop to think, recognise that stress is putting a strain on many aspects of their lives, including relationships. The beneficial effects of following Ayurvedic advice and modifying your lifestyle can be felt so quickly that you will be encouraged to keep trying, and taking medicines which have no unpleasant side-effects, changing your diet and taking regular exercise suddenly do not seem so difficult after all

A full translation of all the Sanskrit texts relating to Ayurveda would fill volumes and volumes and would take a lifetime to understand fully. In this small publication I hope that, helped by thirty years of experience, I have managed to convey the basic rules and ideas of the science. I hope too that I have managed to persuade the reader that this complete system is wholly relevant to modern life and therefore deserving of serious attention.

FURTHER READING

Ananda, Sri, *The Complete Book of Yoga* (Orient Paperbacks), India, 1989.

Baker, Dr Douglas, *Meditation Theory and Practice* (Douglas Baker Publishing), UK, 1985.

Baker, Dr Douglas, *The Jewel in the Lotus* (Douglas Baker Publishing), UK, 1982.

Baker, Dr Douglas, *The Seven Pillars of Ancient Wisdom* (Douglas Baker Publishing), UK, 1982.

Biu, Wang Chi, *The Scientific Outlook of Buddhism* (Buddist Education Foundation), Taiwan, 1985.

Caxton Publishing, *The Encyclopaedia of Herbs and Herbalism*, UK, 1989.

Chopra, Dr Deepak, *Unconditional Life* (Bantam Books), USA, 1992.

Chopra, Dr Deepak, *Quantum Healing* (Bantam Books), USA, 1989.

Chopra, Dr Deepak, *Return of the Rishi* (Houghton Mifflin Co.), USA, 1988.

Dutt, Dr Narain, *Indian Astrology* (Sahni Publications), India, 1996.

Government Department of Languages, *Charaka Samhita – Text Book of Ayurveda* (Government Press), Sri Lanka, 1960.

Government Department of Languages, *Susrutha Samhita – Text book of Surgery* (Government Press), Sri Lanka, 1960.

Government Department of Languages, *Vagbhata Samhita – Text book of Ayurveda by Vagbhata Samhita* (Government Press), Sri Lanka, 1959.

Government Department of Languages, *Madhava Nidana – Text book of Ayurvedic Pathology according to Rishi Madhava* (Government Press), Sri Lanka, 1959.

Hale, Teresa, *The Hale Guide to Good Health* (Kyle Cathie), UK, 1996.

Nagarathna, Dr, Dr Robin Monro and Dr Nagendra, *Yoga for Common Ailments* (Gaia), UK, 1994.

Oriental Medicine (Serinda Publications), UK, 1996.

Narada, The Venerable, *The Buddha and His Teachings* (Buddha Educational Foundation), Taiwan, 1993.

Narada, The Venerable, *The Dhammapada – The Way of Righteousness* (Buddhist Missionary Society), Malaysia, 1978.

Santina, Peter D, *Fundamentals of Buddhism* (Buddhist Educational Foundation), Taiwan, 1984

Shearer, Alistair and Peter Russell, *The Upanishads – Path to Enlightenment, 800BC* (Wildwood House), UK, 1978.

Sivananda Yoga Centre, *The Book of Yoga* (Ebury Press), UK, 1983.

Sumedho, Ajahn, *The Way It Is* (Amaravati Publications), UK, 1989.

Shree, Swami, Puruhit *The Geetha – The Essence of Self-Knowledge* (Faber and Faber), UK, 1978.

Swarupananda, Swami, Srimad *Bhagavad Geetha – Essence of Self Knowledge, 800BC* (Advita Ashram) India, 1909.

Zang, Dr, *Aids and Chinese Medicine* (Keats Publishing), USA, 1995.

AYURVEDIC PRODUCTS FOR COMMON AILMENTS

The following products, used for treating common ailments, are available from Ayurvedic pharmacies (see page 128):

Allergic dermatitis
Eladic (external application oil)

Anaemia
Avipathi Choorna (oral powder)
Dadimadi Ghrita (oral ghee)
Drakshadi Lehya (oral syrup)
Gulguluthikthaka Ghritha (oral ghee)
Kalyanaka Ghrita (oral ghee)
Kishor (oral pills)
Yogaraja (oral pills)

Aphrodisiac
Potentex (external application oil)
Saraswatharishta (oral tonic)

Arthritis
Dashammoola
Rhumarth (external application-massage oil)
Vata Gajendra Singha
Yogaraja

Asthma
Dasamoolarishta (oral tonic)
Dasamoola Rasayana (oral syrup)
Draksha
Goroch (oral pills)
Kanakasava
Kishor (oral pills)
Naradiya Laxi Vilasa
Sithopaladi
Vasaka
Vayu (oral pills)

Bronchial problems
Dadimadi Ghritha (oral ghee)
Vedic Elixir (oral syrup)

Bronchitis
Dasamoolarishta (oral tonic)
Jeerakadyarishta (oral tonic)

Catarrh
Amla 49
Pippaladasava
Rasnadi Choorna (external application powder)
Trikalu

Coitus Reflex (male)
Prolong (external application oil)

Colds and flu
Amla 49
Asana Eladi Thaila (external application oil)
Asana Vilwadi Thaila (external application oil)
Eladi Coconut Oil (external application)
Naradiyalaxmi Vilassa
Nimbamrithadi Castor Oil (oral laxative)
Rasnadi Choorna (external application powder)
Tri Kalu

Constipation
Abhayarishta (oral tonic)
Digesic (oral tablets)
Herbolax
Hing (oral pills)
Sukumara Ghritha (oral ghee)
Triphala

Convalesence
Vedic Elixir (oral syrup)

Cough
Avipathi Choorna (oral powder)
Dasamoola Rasayana (oral syrup)
Goroch (oral pills)
Hing (oral pills)
Jeerakadyarishta (oral tonic)
Vayu (oral pills)
Vilwadi Lehya (oral syrup)

Cystitis
Chandanasava
Immune Cale
Punarnava

Dandruff
Long Locks (external application oil)

Diabetes, non-insulin-dependent
Diabecon
Gulguluthikthaka Kashaya (oral decoction)
Gulguluthikthaka Ghritha (oral ghee)
Kalyanaka Ghritha (oral ghee)
Karela
Kishor (oral pills)

Diarrhoea
Jeerakadyarishta (oral tonic)

Digestion, Poor (*Agni*)
Ashta Choorna (oral powder)
Avipathi Choorna (oral powder)
Dadimadi Ghritha (oral ghee)
Indukantha Ghritha (oral ghee)
KalyanakaGhritha (oral ghee)
Vilwadi Lehya (oral syrup)

Eczema
Eladic (external application oil)
Eladi Coconut Oil (external application)
Eladi Choorna (external application powder)
Kadirarishta
Nimbarishta
Thikthakam Kashaya (oral decoction)

Fainting
Aswagandharishta (oral tonic)
Chandanadi Thaila (external application oil)
Kalyanaka Ghritha (oral ghee)

Fever
Amrutharishta (oral tonic)
Avipathi Choorna (oral powder)
Dasamoola Harithaki (oral syrup)
Goroch (oral pills)
Patadi (oral pills)
Rasnadi Choorna (external application powder)

Flatulence
Digesic (oral tablets)
Gasex
Ramabana

Gaseous stomach
Abhayarishta (oral tonic)
Ashta Choorna (oral powder)
Chandanasava
Dadimadi Ghritha (oral ghee)
Dhanwantharam Kashaya (oral decoction)
Gasex
Ramabana
Sukumaram Ghritha (oral ghee)
Vayu (oral pills)

General tonic
Drakshadi Lehya (oral syrup)

Halitosis
Dasanakanthi Choorna (oral powder)

Hair Loss
Long Locks (external application oil)

Headache
Anui Thaila
Asana Eladi Thaila (external application oil)
Asana Vilwadi Thaila (external application oil)
Ksheerabala Thaila (external application oil)
Neelyadi Oil (external)
Nimbamrithadi Castor Oil (oral laxative)
Rasnadi Choorna (external application powder)
Triphala
Vata Gajendrasingha

Heart conditions
Dasamoolarishta (oral tonic)

High blood pressure
Dashamoola
Sarpaganda

Hyperacidity
Indukantha Ghritha (oral ghee)
Vilwadi Lehya (oral syrup)

Indigestion
Abhayarishta (oral tonic)
Ashta Choorna (oral powder)
Balarishta (oral tonic)
Chiruvilwadi Kashaya (oral decoction)
Digesic (oral tablets)
Goroch (oral pills)
Jeerakadyarishta (oral tonic)
Vilwadi Lehya (oral syrup)

Insect bites
Sathadhowtha Ghritha (external application ghee)

Insomnia
Brahmi
Dashamoola
Kalyanaka Ghritha (oral ghee)
Manas (oral pills)
Mind Cal
Neelyadi oil (external application)

Irritable bowel syndrome (IBS)
Diarex
Isabgol (oral powder)
Musthak
Ramabana
Vilvadi

Itchy scalp
Long Locks (external application oil)

Menopause
Dashamoola
Geriforte
Chandanasava

Menstrual problems
Sukumaram Ghritha (oral ghee)

Nausea
Vilwadi Lehya (oral syrup)

Osteoarthritis
Gulguluthikthaka Ghritha (oral ghee)

Peptic ulcer
Indukantha Ghritha (oral ghee)
Shatavari
Sukumara

Piles
Abhayarishta (oral tonic)
Chiruvilwadi Kashaya (oral decoction)
Dadimadi Ghritha (oral ghee)
Sukumaram Ghritha (oral ghee)

Prostate problems
Chandra Prabha
Shilajit
Uri Care

Rheumatism
Amrutharishta (oral tonic)
Rhumarth (external application-massage oil)

Rheumatoid arthritis
Amrutharishta (oral tonic)
Gulguluthikthaka Ghritha (oral ghee)
Gulguluthikthaka Kashaya (oral decoction)
Kishor (oral pills)
Ksheerabala Thaila (external application oil)
Madhuyastadi Thaila (external application oil)
Nimbamrithadi Castor Oil (oral laxative)
Pinda Thaila (external application-massage oil)
Rasnadi Kashaya (Small) (oral decoction)
Rasnadi Kashaya (Big) (oral decoction)

Rheumatoid arthritis cont…
Rhumarth (external application-massage oil)
Vedic Elixir (oral syrup)

Sexual problems (male)
Potentex (external application oil)
Prolong (external application oil)
Tentex Forte

Sinusitis
Asana Eladi Thaila (external application syrup)
Dasamoola Rasayana (oral syrup)

Skin Diseases
Aragwadhati Kashaya (oral decoction)
Avipathi Choorna (oral powder)
Gulguluthikthaka Ghritha (oral ghee)
Eladi Choorna (external application powder)
Eladi Coconut Oil (external application)
Gulguluthikthaks Ghritha (oral ghee)
Kishor (oral pills)
Thikthakam Kashaya (oral decoction)

Sore throat
Dasamoola Rasayana (oral syrup)

Stomach ache
Indukantha Ghritha (oral ghee)
Vilwadi Lehya (oral syrup)

Stress
Brahmi
Geriforte
Mind Care
Tentex Forte (men)

Urinary problems
Avipathi Choorna (oral powder)
Dhanwanthara Kashaya (oral decoction)
Vedic Elixir (oral syrup)

Vitality, lack of
Amruthaprasa Ghritha (oral ghee)

Ulcers
Aragwadhati Kashaya (oral decoction)
Gulguluthikthaka Ghritha (oral ghee)

GLOSSARY

allergy: hypersensitivity to a substance that causes the body to react internally and externally.

agni: translating as 'fire', the forces which break down the substance consumed, also called metabolism.

ama: an accumulation of toxins, caused by weak *agni*, which circulate throughout the body. They tend to gather in the weak parts of the body and cause disease.

anorexia [nervosa]: a psychological condition characterised by an obsessive desire to lose weight by refusing to eat.

aphrodisiac: anything which arouses sexual desire.

asanas: the 'postures' in yoga.

asceticism: adherence to strict self-discipline and abstention from all forms of pleasure, usually in accordance with religious beliefs and to promote spirituality.

astrology: the study of the movements and relative positions of planets and how they influence human life. It was developed by the ancient Greeks.

athma: the unique, individual 'spirit' which occupies the body and which is transferred to another body on death.

bulimia [nervosa]: a psychological condition characterised by overeating followed by self-induced vomiting or purging.

chakras: circles, without physical manifestation, perceived to be located along the midline of the body, in line with the spinal column.

Charaka Samhita: the principal text written originally in Sanskrit, the codified version of Ayurveda devoted to internal medicine.

chiropractic: the diagnosis and treatment by manipulation of disorders of the spinal column and the joints.

counselling: giving advice; also assistance offered by a professionally trained person in the resolution of problems.

detoxification: thorough external and internal cleansing of the body, recommended as routine treatment, and prior to medical and counselling treatment of specific conditions.

dhaatus: the seven essential tissues which make up the human body (collectively, the *sapta dhaatus*).

dina chariya: a daily programme recommended by Ayurveda for healthy living.

doshas: the three basic constitutional types – *vata*, *pitta* and *kapha* – collectively called the *tridosha*. When they are normal, they are called the three *dhaatus*.

ectomorph: one of the three basic body types (the others being endomorph and mesomorph) – characterised by thinness and weakness.

elements: in ancient and medieval philosophy, the four substances – Air, Fire, Water and Earth – thought to constitute the universe and everything in it.

endomorph: one of the basic body types (the others being ectomorph and mesomorph) – characterised by roundness, fatness and heaviness.

fasting: abstention from all or some kinds of food.

genetics: the study of heredity and inherited characteristics.

geriatrics: the branch of medicine concerned with the treatment of elderly and their diseases.

ghee: butter or milk fat, clarified by boiling and used in Indian cooking.

gunas: characteristics which can be attributed to all matter, organic and inorganic, and to thoughts and ideas. There are twenty.

gynaecology: the branch of medical science concerned with diseases in women, especially those of the genito-urinary tract.

holistic: describes a method of treating a whole person, body, mind, and spirit, rather than just the symptoms of a disorder.

homoeopathy: the treatment of disease with minute doses of medication which would produce in a healthy person symptoms similar to those produced by the disease.

horoscope: a forecast of someone's future based on the relative position of stars and planets at the time of birth.

humours: in medieval philosophy, the four bodily fluids (blood, phlegm, choler and melancholy) thought to determine emotional and physical disposition.

immunity: the ability of an organism to resist disease through the production of antibodies.

Kama Sutra: an ancient Sanskrit treatise on the art of love and sexual technique.

karma: in Hinduism and Buddhism, the principle of retributive justice determining an individual's state of life and based on the cumulative effect of deeds in previous lives. The word also means 'action'.

kundalini: an energy which is believed to travel upwards through the *chakras*, thus promoting spirituality and divine knowledge.

lymph: a colourless fluid, containing chiefly white blood cells, collected from the tissues of the body and transported through the lymphatic system.

mahabbutas: the Sanskrit term for the elements, to which a fifth, Ether, was added by Indian medical teaching.

malas: waste products of the body, of which the principal ones are faeces, urine and sweat.

manthra karma: oral sound therapy used to protect against ghosts and evil spirits.

mantra: a syllable, word or phrase which may be spoken aloud and repeatedly as an aid to meditation.

marmas: energy points in the body where two or more important functions meet.

marma puncture: the technique of inserting a needle into the *marma* points for certain treatments.

marmasthala: the whole area or surface of *marma* points.

meditation: exercising the mind in contemplation, usually by focusing on a thought or an object.

mesomorph: one of the three basic body types (the others being ectomorph and endomorph) - characterised by muscularity and prominent bone structure.

metabolism: the processes that occur in a living organism to maintain life, through the digestion and absorption of nutrients and the breakdown of food eaten.

nirvana: in Buddhism and Hinduism, the final release from the cycle of reincarnation and the effects of *karma*.

obesity: the state of being very fat or overweight.

obstetrics: the branch of medicine concerned with childbirth and the treatment of women before and after childbirth.

oja: the ultimate vital energy which, though it has no physical form, is thought to pervade the system; sometimes referred to as the eighth *dhaatu* or tissue.

ophthalmology: the branch of medicine concerned with the eye and diseases of the eyes.

osteopathy: the treatment of disease through the manipulation of bones and muscles.

otorhinolaryngology: the branch of medicine concerned with the ear, nose and throat and their diseases.

paediatrics: the branch of medical science concerned with children and the treatment of their diseases.

prakruti: a person's original individual constitution, determined by *dosha* type.

panchakarma: internal cleansing which consists of five forms of therapy – induced vomiting, purging, two types of enema, and nasal inhalation. It is designed to prevent or manage disease, and to restore vitality.

pathogens: agents causing disease.

pharmacopeoia: a published list of drugs with instructions for their use.

prana: vital energy which should be allowed to flow unimpeded through the body. It relates to the life or *athma* (spirit) embodied in each living person. *Prana* is seen as having departed from a dead body.

pranayama: the breathing exercises associated with yoga.

proteins: organic compounds broken down to amino acids in the diet and required by the body to make up tissues such as muscles, hair and nails.

purvakarma: pre-detoxification, external cleansing offered to patients before *panchakarma*, and which comprises the application of oil and steam bath therapy.

Rasayana: the branch of Ayurveda concerned with the promotion of rejuvenation.

reincarnation: the rebirth of the soul in a new body.

Rishis: the wise and holy men in ancient India who meditated and acquired the knowledge which was codified as Ayurveda.

samagni: balanced appetite when digestion, absorption and metabolism are functioning efficiently.

Sanskrit: an ancient Indian language and the sacred language of Hinduism; the language in which Ayurveda was written down.

shad rasa: the six basic food tastes identified by Ayurveda – sweet, acidic, salty, pungent, bitter and astringent.

shaanthi karma: oral therapy, which takes the form of a healing blessing, usually offered when the cause of a long-term disorder is unknown, or when someone is dying.

smirti: a force, which might be interpreted as memory or consciousness and which links the different stages of life and maintains individual identity.

snehana karma: massage with oils, similar to aromatherapy.

srothas: channels of circulating fluid which move *doshas*, nutritional matter and waste products around the body.

swedana karma: sweat therapy.

theja: a personal 'aura' of spiritual development.

toxin: a poison produced by a living organism, especially one formed in the body.

Tridosha: the collective term for the three *doshas*.

Tri-Sootra Ayurveda: the collective name for the three components of the knowledge acquired by the *Rishis* – aetiology, symptomatology and medication.

Vedic: relating to the Veda, the ancient, sacred literature of Hinduism.

yoga: a Hindu system of meditation and asceticism whose aim is to bring about reunification with the universal spirit. Dating back more than 2,000 years, it has eight stages, the first four of which have become a popular form of exercise and relaxation in the West.

INDEX

USEFUL ADDRESSES

Dr Godagama's clinics

Ayurvedic Medical Association UK
The Hale Clinic
7 Park Crescent
London W1N 3HE
Tel: 0171 631 0156

Ayurvedic Clinic
322a St Albans Road
Watford
Herts WD2 5PQ
Tel: 01923 246010

Cannon Hill Clinic
16 Cannon Hill
Southgate
London N14 7HD
Tel: 0181 882 2131

Highfield Clinic
Highfield Lane
St. Albans
Herts AL4 0RJ
Tel: 01727 852 992

Holistic Health Centre
66 London Road
Apsley
Hemel Hempstead
Herts HP3 9SD
Tel: 01442 66880

Milton Keynes Ayurvedic Clinic
17 Bromham Mill
Gifferd Park
Milton Keynes
Bucks MK14 5QP
Tel: 01908 617 089

Milton Keynes Orthopaedic Clinic
Blackberry Court
Walnut Tree
Milton Keynes MK7 7BS
Tel: 01908 604 666

Other UK addresses

Ayurvedic Medical Centre
Dr N. Sathiyamoorthy
1079 Garrett Lane
Tooting
London SW17 02N
Tel: 0181 682 3876

Ayurvedic Company of Great Britain
50 Penywern Road
London SW5 9SX
Tel: 0171 370 2255

Maharishi Ayur-Veda Health Centre
21 Clouston Street
Glasgow G20 8QR
Tel: 0141 946 4663

Trancendental Meditation Centre
4 West Newington Place
Edinburgh EH9 1QT
Tel: 0131 668 1649

Ayurvedic Living
PO Box 188
Exeter EX4 5AB
(Will provide help and information on all aspects of Ayurveda: lifestyle, self-help groups and practitioners)

Ayurvedic News
PO Box 188
Exeter EX4 5AB
(Covers Ayurveda in the UK)

Dr Nanda Kumara
Bharatiya Vidya Bhavan
4a Castle Town Road
London W14 9HQ
Tel: 0171 381 3086

Ayurvedic dispensaries

The Nutri Centre
7 Park Crescent
London W1N 3HE
Tel: 0171 436 5122

Maharishi Ayur-Veda Products
Beacon House
Willow Walk
Shelmesdale
Lancashire WN8 6UR

The Himalayan Drug Company
Vedic Medical Hall
6 Chiltern Street
London W1M 1PA0

Australia and New Zealand

Maharishi Ayur-Veda Health Centres
PO Box 81
Bundoora
Victoria 3083
Australia
Tel: (61) 3 9467 4633
Fax: (61) 3 9467 3199

India

Maharishi Ayur-Veda Health Centres
A 214 New Friends Colony
New Delhi 110065
India
Tel: (91) 11 63 27 60
Fax: (91) 11 683 6682

South Africa

Maharishi Ayur-Veda Health Centre
PO Box 5155
Halfway House
1685
South Africa
Tel: (27) 318 1399
Fax: (27) 318 1872

Chiropractic, Homeopathic and Allied Health Service Profession
PO Box 17055
Groenkloof
Pretoria
0027 South Africa
Tel: (27) 12 469 0022

USA

Mapi Inc.
Garden of the Gods Business Park
1115 Elkton Drive Suite 401
Colorado Springs
CO 80907
USA
Tel: (1) 719 260 5500
Fax: (1) 719 260 7400